THE SEVEN CIRCLES

CHELSEY LUGER and THOSH COLLINS

THE

SEVEN

CIRCLES

Indigenous Teachings for Living Well

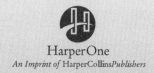

HarperOne

An Imprint of HarperCollinsPublishers

All photos, except as noted, by Thosh Collins or Chelsey Luger, used by permission.

Photograph on page 141 by Angelo Paulos, used by permission.

HarperCollins books may be purchased for educational, business, or sales promotional use. For information, please email the Special Markets Department at SPsales@harpercollins.com.

FIRST EDITION

Designed by Bonni Leon-Berman

Library of Congress Cataloging-in-Publication Data is available upon request.

ISBN 978-0-06-311920-8

22 23 24 25 26   TC   10 9 8 7 6 5 4 3 2 1

For Westyn, Alo, and all Children,

now and Future Generations

CONTENTS

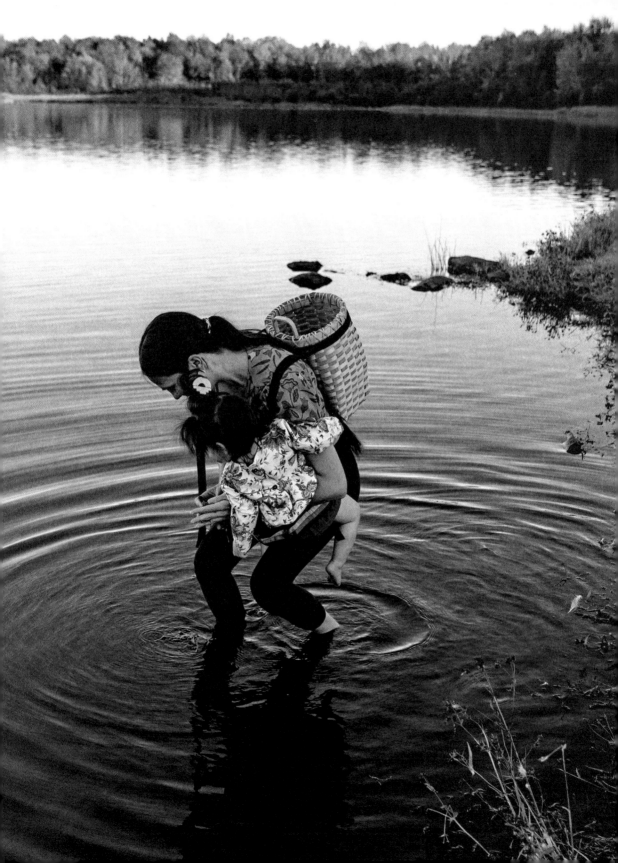

INTRODUCTION

Indigenous traditions are the repository of vast experience and deep insight on achieving balance and harmony. At the time of their first contact with Europeans, the majority of Native American societies had achieved true civilization: they did not abuse the earth, they promoted communal responsibility, they practiced equality in gender relations, and they respected individual freedom.

—Taiaiake Alfred,
Peace, Power, Righteousness: An Indigenous Manifesto

There were ideals and practices in the life of my ancestors that have not been improved upon by the present day civilization; there were in our culture . . . influences that would broaden any life.

—Luther Standing Bear, Land of the Spotted Eagle

Karennenhawi Goodleaf and her daughter, Sakarahkoten, forage for wild herbs and plant medicines.

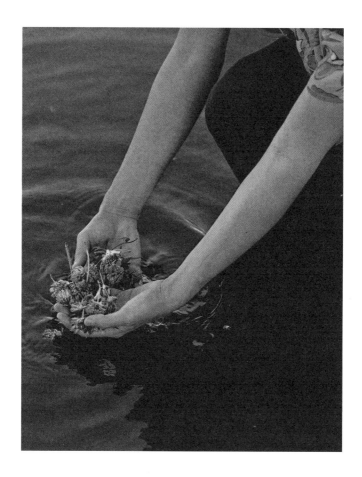

AN INVITATION

On a cool evening in Mohawk territory, a baby girl and her mom are gathering wild herbs. They walk up to the water to make a medicine offering, to reciprocate their harvest. The little girl, familiar with their ritual, digs into her mom's basket to find a bag of tobacco. Her tiny fingers pinch the plant, and she places it gently on the shore. They step into the lake and watch the water ripple outward as they wash the herbs, a reminder that they are closely connected to the world around them. They make a difference. Baby listens while Mom speaks softly to Creator in the original language of the land, acknowledging the water: how it quenches thirst, holds babies in wombs, brings rain and renewal. Together, they are grateful.

Around the Indigenous world, from Aotearoa to Arizona to Alaska, there is one common practice that is shared by nearly all Native people. We begin with gratitude. With each new day, new season, new life, or new endeavor, words and actions of thanks are consciously, generously, deliberately expressed. So, to begin this book, we will honor that.

Today, we are grateful because our life is good. We know who we are, thanks to the ceremonies and teachings that we were raised with. We are proud of who we are, thanks to our peoples' ability to rise above discrimination. We are wellness advocates who genuinely love our work and the people we serve—a joy that is all too uncommon in modern career life. The aim of our work—and this book, by extension—is to help people heal: to make them feel grounded, seen, at ease, and in sync in this complicated, noisy world where it's so easy to get lost. We live by, and have been healed by, the strength and power of our ancestral teachings. So we know that living in balance today, no matter who you are or where you come from, is truly possible.

This book teaches this treasured wisdom—the wellness worldview that our ancestors established and nurtured for good living, and that many in our communities continue to exemplify and practice today. The teachings in this book represent a diverse swath of Indian Country, which reflects the makeup of our family. We are both Native American, but we come from many different places. Chelsey is Anishinaabe from the Turtle Mountain Band of Chippewa, and Hunkpapa and Mniconjou Lakota from the Standing Rock and Cheyenne River Sioux tribes. She grew up on the frozen, wide-open Dakota prairies. Thosh is O'odham, Osage, and Seneca-Cayuga, born and raised on the Salt River Reservation in the desert Southwest, just near the ever-growing metropolis of Phoenix. Our tribal nations are as culturally and linguistically different from one another as Japan and China, or England and France, but our common thread is our Indigenous lineage, which from all sides ties us to the beginning of human history on these lands now known as North America.

Though we come from such different places in Indian Country, we somehow managed to cross paths at precisely the right place and time. (Our people say there are no coincidences, only synchronicity.) In 2013, we were both newly recommitted to personal wellness, we were both on a path to integrating ancestral practices into our healing journeys, and we were both eager to share our miraculously similar vision for Indigenous health with the world. As a writer (Chelsey) and a photographer (Thosh), we made a great team, and we used our skill sets to launch a website and social media platforms that contributed to the existing Indigenous wellness movement by offering a modern, sleek take on everything from tribal food sovereignty to fitness to mindfulness practices.

We got to work right away, and within a few months, we launched a website along with several social media channels. This was a moment in time when people from all fields, industries, and walks of life were just beginning to unlock the potential of online platforms like Twitter, Facebook, and Instagram as educational tools where diverse voices could finally be heard. As mainstream health and wellness platforms grew in popularity online, we anticipated the need for an Indigenous-focused version that would be culturally relevant, social justice oriented, and decolonized. There was nothing like it at the time. We were excited for the opportunity to fight stereotypes and for the world to see Indigenous people at our strongest; but more than that, we were motivated by our communities. We wanted every kid in Native Country to connect their culture to health and to know that not only did they belong in wellness, but they had something to offer to the conversation.

The name we chose for our initiative, Well For Culture, expressed a purpose. Our wellness worldview went beyond the superficial. We wanted to be *well for* our families, *well for* our communities, and *well for* the continuity of our culture. And we hoped to inspire others to do the same.

At first, all of this was just an enjoyable hobby that we focused on after work and between other commitments. We weren't getting paid, but we were having a lot of fun, sharing Indigenous food recipes, shooting "Earth Gym" compilations for YouTube, and writing blog posts like "Which Mocs Should You Rock for Your Workout?" But before we knew it, Well For Culture took on a life of its own, and it became our full-time job. The calls came rolling in, so we began to travel all over—from Indigenous community centers, to elite universities, to Nike world headquarters—to share workshops about Indigenous healthy lifestyles. We haven't stopped since.

After a few years of teaching, learning, and refining as we went, we formalized our wellness methodology by creating a new, unique model: a visual healing tool that is interconnected, dynamic, and cyclical—not stagnant, rigid, or linear. It is called the *Seven Circles of Wellness*, and it includes movement, land, community, ceremony, sacred space, sleep, and food. These are all the aspects of healthy lifestyles that a person needs to live in balance. These are all the areas of living that our ancestors so brilliantly mastered. These circles are what we all need to incorporate into our wellness journeys today.

Now, we are honored by the opportunity to share the Seven Circles of Wellness with you. This book is an invitation. We welcome you to build strength, to heal, and to honor your whole self through Indigenous wellness philosophies and practices.

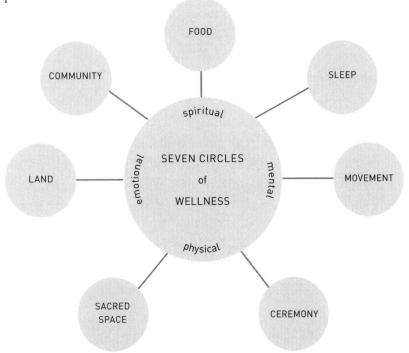

We find it fascinating, and truly a missed opportunity, that most Americans today are familiar with culturally specific health-oriented practices from many other parts of the world—be it hygge from Denmark, feng shui from China, or yoga from India—but know nothing of the ancient wellness teachings from the land on which they stand. This ignorance was no accident. Indigenous voices have been shut out and silenced from all parts of the American story. Now, we are speaking up and inserting ourselves into the health and wellness conversation, right where we belong. We know that settler colonialism is the root of many of the health challenges that people face today—Indigenous or not—and that understanding this will help people heal. We also know that health through the Indigenous lens will be refreshing and uplifting for many people. The wellness industry is dominated by limited ideas that prioritize physical appearance, consumerism, and youth. We offer tools for people of all backgrounds to connect to a wellness practice that is more than skin deep.

We want you to know that the knowledge presented here is not "purely" anything. We do not claim to be staunchly traditionalist, nor do we pretend to lead strictly ancestral lifestyles. We are not anti-Western medicine, we are not anti-technology, and we are certainly not antiscience. We arrived at our health perspective by studying Indigenous history to see how our ancestors lived, by being raised within our respective Indigenous communities, by spending time with elders and knowledge keepers, by trial and error, by poring over academic papers, by integrating perspectives from our ceremonial backgrounds, and by consulting with health resources outside of our culture. From there, we have figured out how to incorporate each of these Seven Circles into our modern lifestyles in mindful, effective ways. We hope that what we share with you on the following pages will bring you the balance and comfort that it has brought to us.

We echo the sentiment of Wilma Mankiller, a late great chief of the Cherokee Nation, who once wrote that she "made a conscious choice to lead a meaningful life by building on the positive attributes of [her] communities instead of focusing only on the daunting set of economic and social problems."[1] We see ourselves as doing the same. This book is a way for us to honor the teachings that our ancestors worked tirelessly to pass on. It is a celebration of Indigenous ideas, a gift to those who will listen, and a bold refusal to leave good health in the past. As Mankiller's friend, feminist Gloria Steinem, wrote of Indigenous knowledge, "these lifeways could be the wheels that will carry us all."[2]

The Legacy of Our Ancestors

As Indigenous people, we are the grandchildren of survivors. Our ancestors were people of mighty courage, daunting intelligence, physical prowess, and spiritual strength. We know this because they managed to survive a genocide that not many people understand the severity of but that changed the course of human history and health forever. Colonization began five hundred years ago, and it hasn't yet ended. Led by the amoral guidance of the Doctrine of Discovery and Manifest Destiny, Europeans stopped at nothing to take life, land, and livelihood from our people. Their invasion initiated widespread ecological disruption and led to the destruction of the once-symbiotic relationship between human, plant, and animal populations. They imposed an industrial, capitalist economy that made it impossible for most people today—Native or not—to live in a way that honors the health of the people or the planet. In 1492, somewhere between twenty million and one hundred million Indigenous people lived in North America. By 1900, only two hundred thousand were left. Our ancestors are survivors.

This devastating history is recent and raw. Our people still reel from its effects. But here we are today, still grateful, because our tribal nations remained intact despite oppressive government programs that were explicitly designed to destroy our communities and kill our culture; because our spiritual practices survived, even though our dances and ceremonies were illegal until 1978; because our grandparents outlasted the horrors of abusive, assimilative boarding schools and came together to work hard and raise families on our reservations; because our strong-willed parents made good lives for us and protected us as best they could, despite the sudden prevalence of addiction, disease, poverty, and other hardships commonly faced in America today.

Life hasn't always been so good for either of us, and struggles continue to weave themselves in and out of our stories. For us, wellness is not a perfect state of being; it is a state of preparedness for the inevitable hardships in life. It is a toolkit for steadiness. We have both narrowly escaped paths of addiction. We have both struggled to learn to survive financially in this cutthroat world. We have both been through unhealthy relationships and periods of low self-worth. We have battled anxiety, depression, and chronic stress. We have both lost close relatives, friends, and loved ones to modern-day ills like diabetes, heart disease, addiction, suicide, and accidental death. We have seen that poor health outcomes are not only worrisome, but life threatening. We intentionally continue our healing journeys because we are never above the risk of falling. We do our wellness work in the names of those who have gone too soon. We honor them by striving every day to be strong and sturdy in body, mind, and spirit. Everyone has been hurt by colonialism. These health issues plague not only Indian Country, but the world. Likewise, everyone must heal.

We are relieved to say that today, we have seized many of our opportunities to heal. We have abandoned lifestyle patterns that did not serve us and replaced them with habits that make us whole. We have learned to keep a sacred circle of healthy relationships, while setting firm boundaries with people, places, and substances that are harmful. We have remembered and revitalized ancestral teachings in relation to food, plant medicine, parenting, and community, and we do our best to live by these. We are sober, we are active, and we often wake up with clear minds and good hearts, ready to make the most of each day. There are hard times, and there are heartbreaking phone calls from back home. There are nights of no sleep with our babies, and there are always work and stress. But for the most part, we find ourselves thriving and living well, knowing where to go and what to do when we start to feel ourselves fall.

To hear that we are a thriving Native family may come as a surprise, because the mainstream media relentlessly perpetuates stereotypes about us, making a nightly news spectacle of our alleged downtroddenness. But the truth is, over the past few generations, Native people have been recovering en masse from historical trauma, leading full and happy lives and succeeding in every way imaginable, from education, to career, to family life. Our thriving is not *despite* our culture, but *because of* our culture. This may come as a double surprise, because just as modern media have stereotyped us, popular history has all but erased Indigenous voices, knowledge, philosophies, worldviews, and contributions from the pages of textbooks. Not only do most Americans not understand the breadth of knowledge that Indigenous culture has to offer, many Indigenous people ourselves have not been afforded the opportunity to simply be proud of our brilliance. But this is changing.

Our populations have continued to rebound, our leaders are creating space for cultural regeneration, our media makers are erasing stereotypes, our teachers are reintegrating Indigenous languages, our artists are showing the world our beauty, while our tribal governments (more than five hundred of them) are asserting our sovereignty. Native children today are growing up healthy, happy, and whole, armed with the richness of their identity. We make a point to emphasize this because the negative side of Native life has been overexploited. Our struggle exists, sure, but it is not our complete story. In order to understand health and wellness from an Indigenous perspective, one must recognize and respect the positive aspects of Native culture, noting the remarkable amount of healing that our people have done. If we can continue to stand in our power after five hundred years of colonial abuses, then perhaps we indeed have something to teach the world in the way of conjuring resilience.

This mental, physical, emotional, and spiritual strength-building is where our work focuses. As full-time wellness advocates, we share educational tools online and travel the world to teach, learn, and present techniques for healing and living well. We have worked with corporations like Nike and Google; we have spoken before academic audiences at Johns Hopkins, Stanford, and Dartmouth; we have been featured by media outlets like BBC World News and the *New York Times*. Most important, we have done this work hand-in-hand, in alignment and in solidarity with our peers at tribal colleges, reservation wellness centers, suicide prevention programs, youth councils, Indian Health Service offices, Indigenous nonprofits, and all other Native-led efforts in this area of health reclamation.

Over the course of a decade in wellness work, we have built lasting bonds with the Indigenous people and nations who have hosted us. Getting to know the diversity of Indian Country in a deeper way, beyond the communities we were raised in, has been the honor of our lives. With our friends and colleagues by our sides and as our guides, we have dodged swarms of bees in the wave-patterned canyons of the Navajo Nation, and we have tasted the tart, wild strawberries that line the gravel roads where kids in Bad River ride their bikes. We have smelled the sacred fires that burn in the grand timber longhouses on the Salish coast, and we have feasted on roots, berries, and smoked wild game served with stunning formality by the women of the Great Basin. From the Passamaquoddy in Maine to the Pechanga in Southern California, each and every tribal nation today bursts with unique character and cultural dynamism. These places should be seen first and foremost for their gifts, their power, their beauty, and their knowledge, not for their traumas or hardships. Allies often ask us: How can we help Indian Country? We say: You cannot help us. You can learn from us.

We know this from experience. When we are invited to work in tribal communities, we are asked to teach, but we walk away having learned. We are educated by the elders who share the science of their sacred medicines. We are floored by the children who come to us with the most thought-provoking questions. We are wellness trainers, but we do not consider ourselves experts who can swoop in and bring quick, straightforward fixes to solve health disparities, as those with "white savior" mentalities have a history of doing in our communities. We are humbled to stand before doctors, social workers, educators, and parents who are the descendants of chiefs, clan mothers, medicine people, and warriors. They have suffered unfathomable losses, they face ongoing struggles of their own, but they still get out of bed every day committed to making life better for their children. This undying love for our future generations and steadfast focus on intergenerational healing is the heart of Indigenous wellness today. We have seen it.

Defining Indigenous Wellness

To be clear, the Seven Circles of Wellness is rooted in ancestral wisdom and pulls from an intertribal array of knowledge, but it is not an ancient model itself. Many elders and leaders in the public health world have given it their blessing when they have seen it, though it is not universally acknowledged or practiced among all Indigenous groups. There is no such thing as a singular, pan-Indian perspective on health (or on anything else, for that matter). This is a new model, created by us: two individuals who come from intertribal backgrounds. We have connected the dots between our specific cultural upbringings, spiritual worldviews, and modern health needs to create a wellness model that all people can use. Throughout this book, we heavily reference Lakota, Ojibwe, O'odham, and Haudenosaunee teachings because these are the nations we come from, and so we have inevitably learned more from these cultural perspectives. All Indigenous cultures carry wellness teachings, and all Indigenous people have our own ways of looking at wellness—this one is ours. Our model integrates concepts that are common in the Indigenous world, like interconnectedness, balance, healing, and gratitude, but it does not claim to comprehensively include all Indigenous perspectives on health, as this would be impossible. As the makers of it, we do our best to represent our communities and families, but we do not speak *for* them. All inadequacies or shortcomings are our own.

Our goal is to acknowledge, uplift, and shine light on Indigenous health knowledge in a way that does not minimize its breadth. Our perspective on Indigenous health is far from the only one. Through this resource, we hope to help people unlearn any stereotypical narratives. Indigenous people are dynamic and diverse, not savage, not primitive, not a monolith, not mystical, and not anything else that dehumanizes us. Although for lack of better options we use broad terms like "Indigenous wellness" or "the Indigenous approach," we also recognize that there is no single way to define Indigenous perspectives on anything.

Guidelines, Not Rules: A Sustainable Approach

Wellness is a multibillion-dollar industry. Every day, a new guru or health coach is pitching fad diets and fitness trends as the be-all and end-all solution to our problems. And yet, these trends that we are so urgently pushed to adapt always end up fading. With so many different experts pulling us in different directions, it might feel impossible to make sense of it all, and frustratingly confusing to figure out how to begin a health journey. Indigenous knowledge is the opposite of trend. It is both futuristic and ancient, perfectly adaptable to the present. It is exactly what is needed to counter mainstream wellness culture, which capitalizes on both illness and sickness, revolves around fads, and puts ethics aside to pitch products for profit.

Just as Indigenous communities have always valued environmental sustainability by taking care of the land, water, and resources for future generations, we aim for longevity and sustainability in wellness. We emphasize nurturing a steady flow of interconnectedness and balance, rather than reaching a state of ultimate perfection. We offer guidelines, not rules, that allow for constant learning and adjustment, as opposed to precise instructions with a specific desired outcome. The Seven Circles of Wellness are the antithesis to extreme diet and exercise plans. More than trying to physically transform your body, we want to help expand your mind and heart. We want all people to feel welcome, accepted, and included in the wellness space, one that has historically excluded many people, especially those from marginalized communities. We hope to take away the shame so that you can feel the same sense of security and unconditional love that we have felt when learning from our elders.

We feel confident that the Seven Circles of Wellness is a wonderfully refreshing way of approaching health and wellness, and while we certainly hope that you, the reader, gets something great out of it, we want you to know that it's okay if you don't agree with everything we say, if you walk away not viewing health exactly as we view it, or if you connect to only bits and pieces of our offering. This might seem odd, considering that most wellness advocates are very adamant that their way is the best way. But proselytism has never been the way for Native people. Our ancestors, who were deeply spiritual but not "religious," believed in the fundamental human right to pray, live, and believe in whatever one chose, and we still uphold this commitment to freedom of thought today. It goes beyond religion and spirituality and permeates our perspectives on daily life and, indeed, approaches to health. Indigenous culture is nonjudgmental, nonpreachy, and open minded. We approach wellness with that mentality. You are more than welcome to take or leave any aspect of the concepts that we present to you. You may combine our ideas with any preexisting set of beliefs and practices that you follow. The only way to go wrong in wellness is to exploit, to appropriate, or to demonstrate ignorance about or disrespect to another group or culture. Those errors aside, there are no mistakes on your journey to better health.

When viewed through the Indigenous lens, health and wellness can become so much more than an extracurricular activity or a method of fixing oneself. Western fitness culture centers thin, white, able, young bodies and has led us all to believe that seeking wellness is materialistic, exclusive, and elitist at its core. This is probably why the word "wellness" prompts eye-rolls for so many people. Our approach works for those who are burned out on gimmicks. We integrate family and community, we acknowledge barriers to access, we encourage cultural authenticity, and we include all ages, proving that self-healing is not selfish, because it makes an impact on the world around you.

We know that the Indigenous people who are reading this book will be excited to find a wellness resource that appropriately acknowledges the real root of most health problems in America today: settler colonialism. We encourage all readers to duly remember that settler colonialism is not an isolated system that only affected Native people in the past. It is an ongoing process that continues to harm the health and livelihood of all exploited lands today and the people who live on them. Engaging with Indigenous wellness and reintegrating Indigenous teachings into your health worldview is a powerful way to begin to unlearn many of the harmful, normalized habits that are now prevalent in everyday American life.

By the end of this book, you will feel comfortable applying the Seven Circles of Wellness to your own life, in your own way. After learning from it, you will feel confident in your ability to seek balance, as opposed to perfection, in your wellness journey. In Anishinaabe culture, there is a concept called *mino bima-diizawin*, the good life. In Lakota culture, there is walking the *canku luta*, or the red road. In O'odham culture, people aim for *s-doakag*, walking in a good way. You can probably find a powerful phrase like this in any one of the thousands of Indigenous languages that are spoken around the world. Our elders teach that this "good life" is waiting for you to return to, whenever you are ready: no judgment, no questions asked, and no timeline. Whether this book becomes a tattered and well-loved companion on your bedside table or ends up collecting dust on your bookshelf, know that the Seven Circles of Wellness will always be there, ready to help you return to balance.

It is not only our honor, but also our role and our duty to contribute this Indigenous perspective to the wellness world at large. We are so excited for all people to learn about Indigenous cultures through this lens of wellness and health. We pray that all readers benefit in some way, big or small, from accepting these powerful lifestyle practices into daily life. Through this, we honor the healing wisdom that our ancestors carried on, against all odds, through many generations, and passed down to us so that we may share with you. The sacred cycle of Indigenous culture continues to thrive and grow. So here we are today, grateful.

An Exercise—Find Your Power

> Wakan-Tanka [Great Spirit] puts natural power inside of each person when they are born . . . This is a gift Wakan-Tanka gives freely to us.
>
> —*Frank Fools Crow, from* Fools Crow: Wisdom and Power

Find a seat on the ground, or hold a stone in your hand, or plant your feet firmly on the floor. The earth, our ancestors teach, is where we go to be connected.

Visualize an exchange of energy between you and the ground that is holding you up. You are connected. You are rooted. You are strong.

Now, examine your hands. They tell a story of both ancestry and individuality. On your palms are bloodlines that tie you to your collective identity. And yet, close observation of every intricate groove, crease, and fingerprint reminds you that you are unique. Embrace your ancestry and your individuality. Give yourself permission to use your hands to carry the good and the strength that you have inherited. Give yourself permission to brush off, with your hands, the things you have inherited that you do not wish to carry.

Now, rub the palms of your hands together. Start slow, then pick up speed. After about twenty seconds, when you feel the heat of their friction, hover your hands in front of your face without touching your skin. Close your eyes as you do this. What do you feel?

The heat from the friction you created is a physical manifestation of the spiritual energy that flows throughout your body, connecting you to the great Creator. This is your power. You were born with it, and you will die with it. No one can take this away from you, no matter how hard they try. No matter what you have been through, you have always held your power. It is important that you remember this. Take time to access it every so often. Teach others to find theirs as well.

Everyone can harness their power and build it. Like a fire, it needs to be fed to grow. You might already be subconsciously accessing this power in your everyday life. Some use it to remind themselves of their own worth and strength. Others use it to help them achieve visionary ideas. Athletes use it for sport and movement. Artists use it to paint, shape, and build. Parents use it for caregiving. Musicians use it to create sound. Doctors use it for healing. You may use it however you choose.

In our ancestors' time, everyone understood that they had the power within them to do good things, to be a good person, and to live a good life. Dominant culture has led many of us to stray from this self-empowerment. You are not weak or broken. You are strong, and you can heal. Know your own power.

TURNING YOUR MINDSET TOWARD INDIGENOUS WELLNESS: FOUNDATIONAL CONCEPTS, THEORIES, AND SUGGESTIONS

⊕ The Medicine Wheel ⊕

The medicine wheel is an ancient symbol—a circle divided into four parts, usually red, black, yellow, and white—that symbolizes balance, interconnectedness, and gratitude for all things that bring us life. It comes from the Great Plains region but is recognized by Indigenous people all over the world. Today in Indian Country, you will see medicine wheels created in quillwork on regalia, depicted on educational pamphlets, worn with permanent pride on tattoo art, incorporated into logos for tribal businesses, and even memorialized on the earth itself. In Cree territory (Alberta, Canada), there is a massive stone monument of the medicine wheel that predates the pyramids of Giza in Egypt.

There are countless ways to interpret the medicine wheel. Like most Indigenous knowledge, it is not a rigid concept. One common interpretation is that each quadrant represents the four universal parts of existence: mental, physical, emotional, and spiritual. They also represent the four cardinal directions and the life-giving forces that come from each of those directions. For example, black often symbolizes the west, which is where the Thunder Beings come from, which bring life in the form of rain, renewal, clarity, water, fire, energy, and opportunity.

The medicine wheel is a powerful educational tool that continues to inform many Indigenous peoples' understandings of how to live a good, healthy, balanced life. It has been a key piece of our own understandings of health and healing from the time that we were children—particularly Chelsey, who grew up in Lakota culture, where the medicine wheel is prominent. A basic understanding of the medicine wheel will help in understanding the Seven Circles of Wellness. It is because of the medicine wheel, and other Indigenous symbols like it, that we have come to understand health through this lens of interconnectedness and balance. It could be said that there is a medicine wheel within each of the Seven Circles, because each of them have mental, physical, spiritual, and emotional facets.

Within each chapter of this book, you will find a section (for example, "Move-ment Medicine Wheel") that clearly explains each mental, physical, spiritual, and emotional aspect of the circle, as it is important to acknowledge the holistic and far-reaching healing that can happen by incorporating each circle into your life.

Fools Crow's Hollow Bone Theory

One can visualize one's own ability to heal and find power within by seeing oneself as a hollow bone. Frank Fools Crow was a Lakota medicine man and Sun Dance chief who lived from 1890 to 1989. He was alive during a long and painful era when Lakota ceremonies were illegal, and he was instrumental in keeping them alive and revitalizing them. He played a big role in helping thousands of Lakota people main-tain and reclaim their spiritual beliefs throughout those decades. (Chelsey's father is one person who began attending Fools Crow's Sun Dance after a childhood of being raised in the Catholic Church, so even though we have never personally met Fools Crow, he is an elder-ancestor who has played a big role in shaping our world-view and making this book possible.) Through Fools Crow's autobiography and through the oral tradition, we are able to keep learning from him today. One of his most profound teachings is what we refer to as the *hollow bone theory*.

Fools Crow reminds us that even though he was highly regarded as a healer and medicine man, he saw himself as an *ikceya wicasa*—a common man. Like everyone else, he had to put effort into living a certain lifestyle in order to con-jure up and maintain his ability to help and heal others. He said, "Anyone who is willing to live the life I have led can do the things I do." He viewed himself, and other medicine people, as "hollow bones" that Wakan-Tanka (the Great Spirit), *tunksasila* (Grandfather Creator), and other spirit helpers work in and through. Furthermore, he said that all people, not just medicine people, can be hollow bones. In other words, they may live in a way that allows them to be well and to serve others. Being a hollow bone means being open to receiving, learning, and taking in good teachings and good ways of life, and then taking on the respon-sibility of passing those good ways of life on to others.[3]

Today in seeking wellness, we ask ourselves, what exactly were those habits and ways of being that someone like Fools Crow followed in his own life? Of his own lifestyle, he shares:

> I do not argue, do not fight, do not hate, do not gossip, and I have never said a swear word. I have not taken advantage of anyone. I have not charged for my curing, healing, or advice, although I have accepted the gifts of gratitude people have brought to me. I have never touched alcohol or drugs. Wakan-Tanka (the Great Spirit) can take me higher than any drug ever could.[4]

Fools Crow lived this way not because he was forced to, and certainly not because there is a spirituality rulebook that says a person has to be this way. He did this because he chose to. We have observed this lifestyle of self-discipline and attitude of humility while reading about Fools Crow, but also by observing, reading about, and learning from other Indigenous leaders and healers past and present. We believe that in conjunction with viewing oneself as a hollow bone who is open to receiving and learning at all times, one can intentionally self-determine a clear set of values and behavioral standards and turn one's life toward wellness.

Standing Bear's Law of Self-Mastery

Ancestral teachings frequently purport what Luther Standing Bear, a well-known Lakota writer and advocate who lived around the same time as Fools Crow, has called the *law of self-mastery*. Self-mastery is the ability of an adult to demonstrate measured thinking, to be careful with words, to make thoughtful decisions, and to remain level-headed under any circumstance. This involves a great deal of discipline, hard work, and patience. Standing Bear described self-mastery as a "powerful agent" that gives a person an opportunity to develop into a "true human." When practiced, it helps us live in balance as individuals, and it also positively impacts our communities. Standing Bear wrote, "True civilization lies in the dominance of self and not in the dominance of other men."[5]

Living as we do in the world of digital noise, constant emails, busy urban life, and the twenty-four-hour news cycle, we are unwittingly riding an unending emotional rollercoaster that demands quick reactions and immediate responses. Those who demonstrate controversy, fast-thinking, and loudness are rewarded with more attention and more opportunities, and so the cycle continues. Today, in seeking balance, we must strive to radically remove ourselves from this pattern. Attention to all aspects of the Seven Circles of Wellness will help us to arrive at this place of self-control and self-awareness.

Of note, Standing Bear emphasized that this self-mastery should always be voluntary, not imposed. Keep this in mind as you continue to read this book. Remind yourself that no one is forcing you to be well, to be healthy, or to live in balance. You have chosen this path for yourself. This advice will also prove useful if you find yourself frustrated with or concerned about a loved one who is suffering from poor health and is unwilling or unable to change. It is good to offer support and encouragement to another person on their wellness journey, but know that any attempt to force it will be fruitless. Self-mastery must come from within.

Systemic Inequity and Social Determinants of Health

In spite of the many revelatory Indigenous methodologies for finding, creating, and asserting our own inner power, we must also acknowledge the myriad barriers to health that many people currently face. A report published by the National Academies of Sciences defines *health inequities* as systematic differences in the opportunities groups have to achieve optimal health, leading to unfair and avoidable differences in health outcomes.[6] The report says that the root cause of health inequity is the "unequal allocation of power and resources—including goods, services, and societal attention—which manifest in unequal social, economic, and environmental conditions, also called the social determinants of health." An individual's health status is only partially determined by behavior and choice, yet largely dependent upon an interplay of structures, systems, and community-wide factors like violence, historic injustices, poverty, unemployment, policies, and resulting norms, and that the distribution of power and resources varies widely across lines of race, gender, class, sexual orientation, gender expression, and other dimensions of individual and group identity.[7] Simply put, the pursuit of health is not a fair game.

As two people who grew up seeing widespread health disparities among our own families and communities, we have deep compassion for this. Thosh's community, Salt River, became well-known in the 1990s for having the highest rates of diabetes in the world, and Chelsey's community, Standing Rock, has famously battled environmental racism with the conflict over the Dakota Access Pipeline. In addition to these systemic community challenges that we have been a part of, we have seen no end to health struggles in our own families. We wholeheartedly empathize with, sympathize with, and respect the barriers to approaching a balanced lifestyle that so many people face.

We continue to face some of these barriers as well, but we also acknowledge our privilege in not experiencing or understanding others. We encourage all readers to do the same: acknowledge and learn to identify both your barriers and your privilege. Remember to avoid judging or shaming yourself or others when it comes to health. Until we all recognize and respect these inequities, we cannot emerge from them.

Acknowledgment of underlying and overarching health disparities is a defining feature of the Indigenous wellness mentality. Mainstream American fitness culture pitches rhetoric that constantly oversimplifies the health process, calling everything a "choice," urging people to get "motivated" and to get their "priorities" straight. Our intention is to move away from this binary thinking and oversimplification, acknowledging the complexity in all aspects of the wellness journey, which is one of many reasons that we do not offer specific instructions or rules throughout this book. We want to remind each of you, our readers, that you do not need to do every single thing that we suggest or promote; instead, you are free to pull from our suggestions whatever you are able to access and whatever may serve you, wherever you are in your journey.

Trauma-Informed and Healing-Centered

Trauma is a common barrier to wellness that must be acknowledged by all wellness practitioners and seekers. When we recognize, respect, and learn to appropriately respond to trauma, we become *trauma-informed*. This approach can make all the difference in people understanding, and in helping people understand, why the things they have been through and the way they have been treated has led to certain behavioral patterns or hardships. Being trauma-aware and approaching trauma with a compassionate, empathetic perspective can help everyone to better grasp and appreciate both the struggles and the resilience that exist within themselves, their families, their friendships, and their community.

Traumatic experiences can overwhelm an individual's capacity to cope. Trauma can be caused by an extreme form of social adversity. This can include single-incident trauma, for example, an incident of assault; complex or repetitive trauma, such as ongoing abuse or domestic violence; developmental trauma, including exposure to neglect or abandonment as an infant or child; intergenerational trauma, which is the psychological or emotional effects of living with a trauma survivor; or historical trauma, which is a cumulative psychological and emotional wounding that spans generations and stems from a collective group trauma, such as genocide, colonialism, slavery, or war.[8]

We know that trauma can be inherited in a psychosocial context, and now, some scientists are further studying the concept of intergenerational trauma. Some epigenetic studies have suggested that trauma can actually transform the expression of our genes and can be passed down to our children biologically. These conclusions remain hotly debated in the scientific community.[9] But if there is truth to this, we can infer that if trauma can be inherited, so too can resilience. So although it is critical to be able to recognize and respect trauma, we must be careful to not allow trauma to define the fate or experiences of ourselves or others. That is why it is equally important to move beyond being trauma-informed and into being *healing-centered*.

Healing-centered approaches to finding well-being are based on strength, collectively oriented, and embrace the gifts that are inherent in diverse cultural upbringings and perspectives.[10] The Native Wellness Institute is a nonprofit organization that has been doing healing work in Indigenous communities for decades. Jillene Joseph (Aaniiih), its executive director, lives by this ethos: "Where there has been trauma, healing is the answer." We view the Seven Circles of Wellness, and indeed the concept of Indigenous wellness, as a healing-centered approach. In our work, we are moving beyond the question of "What happened to you?" and further asking, "What is right with you? What are your gifts? What are the beneficial, beautiful, and healing aspects of your culture, family, and community that you have experienced and inherited?" From there, anyone can go beyond a state of responding to trauma and can indeed seek happiness, optimal health, and the same wholeness and joy that others dream possible.

Audre Lorde, a Black civil rights activist and feminist, said, "Caring for myself is not self-indulgence. It is self-preservation. And that is an act of political warfare."[11] Caring for yourself might be your way of breaking intergenerational cycles of trauma, and healing yourself will help in healing your family and community. Healthy people make healthy families, healthy families make healthy communities, and healthy communities make healthy tribal nations and indeed a better world.

THE "TAKE ACTION" SECTIONS: LEARN, ENGAGE, OPTIMIZE

Acknowledging that everyone who is coming to this book is at a very different place in life, living in very different circumstances, and with very different needs and objectives in mind, we offer action steps at the end of each chapter that provide some structure for your wellness journey, while still remaining malleable and respectful of your individuality. Within the "Take Action" sections are three categories: Learn, Engage, and Optimize. Generally speaking, there are no precise "levels" to Indigenous wellness. It's not as simple as the standard model of *beginner, intermediate, advanced*. Rather, *learn, engage, optimize* is a constant cycle of growth, and these processes overlap.

Here's more on these categories within each circle:

LEARN: You have just begun to *learn* about how this circle contributes to your wellness, or, you have just begun to learn the Indigenous perspective on this circle, which might be quite different from your prior understanding of it. The "Learn" category gives you ideas about what you might learn in order to engage.

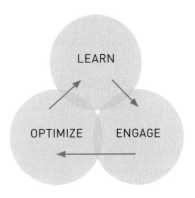

As opposed to the linear nature of "stages" or "levels" in your wellness journey, Learn, Engage, and Optimize are cyclical and ever moving.

ENGAGE: You are now ready to *engage* with this circle and are beginning to consciously use the concepts within it in your daily life and wellness practice. You are figuring out how to apply this circle to your life in a way that makes sense for you and your loved ones. You are experimenting, creating new habits, trying new things, and taking healthy risks.

OPTIMIZE: At this stage, you have learned a lot about this circle and have been fully engaged with a practice within it for some time. You are now *optimizing* your practice, noticing its benefits, thriving, and feeling confident. You are aware of how this circle contributes to your balanced lifestyle as a whole, and you are mentoring and teaching others about how to apply this circle in their lives.

You aren't done after "Optimize." The journey continues. You now return to "Learn." What we have realized through our personal wellness experiences is that whenever we have achieved a sense of thriving in one area, we begin to realize how much we still do not know. It's similar to the conclusion of a scientific study—there are no final "answers," only recommendations for further research. The more you know, the more you know you need to know. That is why the "Optimize" category always circles back to "Learn" once again. But by the time you circle back to learning, you won't need this book anymore to guide your questioning. You will be an informed agent of change who knows what to ask and where to go. Following that, your "Engage" process will also evolve, as will your return to a new state of optimization. The learning, engaging, and optimizing will be a lifelong, cyclical process.

The Constant Ebb and Flow of Balance

Balance is not a perfect state of being that one achieves. It requires a constant returning-to. Day by day, season by season, and year by year, you will continue to flow in and out of connection with each of the Seven Circles of Wellness. At different stages in life, or even from one day to the next, you will be thriving in certain circles, while perhaps neglecting others. Here are a few scenarios of what your Seven Circles may look like from one stage of life to the next.

Scenario 1: Here, you are forty years old. You haven't been doing much with the *movement* circle lately because you suffered a back injury, so exercise has been painful and difficult (so the circle is small in the illustration). Because of the pain, your *sleep* has suffered as well. However, you are very strong in *ceremony* because you have been integrating meditation and mindful breathwork into your daily life, which has been a very helpful tool for stress relief and mental clarity. You have also been intentional about taking your breathwork outdoors, even integrating it into your gardening, so your connection to *land* is also strong. Your *sacred space* circle is a bit smaller because you are having trouble keeping your home clean with several kids in the house. But on the positive side, your home is a comfortable and safe place for your family, so this circle is medium-sized. *Community*, which includes family, is currently shining brightly—you are in the throes of raising your three children. You are an attentive, loving parent, and you consistently take your kids to activities, community gatherings, and to visit their relatives. *Food* is a circle that has suffered for some time, but your hard work in this area is beginning to bring healing. Although you haven't been able to sever your ties with soda, a key player in your sugar addiction, you

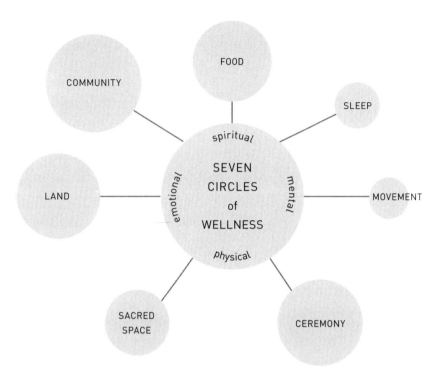

An example of a Seven Circles of Wellness mind-map, which helps you express and visualize what a balanced life might look like for you.

have been growing vegetables in your garden, you are prioritizing home-cooked meals (as opposed to take-out or fast food), and you are remembering to give thanks for your food with every meal.

Scenario 2: Many years later, you are an elder, and your circles look different at this stage in your life. **Food** is thriving more than ever before, as you have continued to grow and harvest your own corn, squash, and beans for many years. You have become a seed keeper who is available to guide others when they have questions about food sovereignty. You are an early riser who loves to greet the sun each morning, and you like to go for a long walk before you begin your other tasks of the day, so your **sleep** and **movement** circles are both very strong as well. **Ceremony** and **community** are smaller circles nowadays. Your kids are

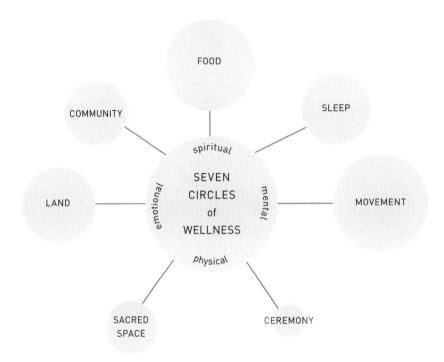

grown up and out of the home, and you have been out of the loop with attending community gatherings, though you would like to get back into it soon, as you long for the good feelings that come with human connection. **Sacred space** is also smaller, because as you get older, you find yourself growing sentimental and having a hard time decluttering your home and letting go of odds and ends that are not of use to you anymore. But recently, you have been intentionally reconnecting to **land** by going on drives to visit sacred sites and see the beautiful scenery around your homelands that you hadn't been to in some time. It feels good to spend time with these places and to remember why they are special to you.

Where Are You Thriving Now?

Imbalance will always be part of a balanced life. Our hope is that in accepting this, you feel a sense of progress and flow already in place, rather than a sense that you are starting your wellness journey from nothing. Engaging with the Seven Circles

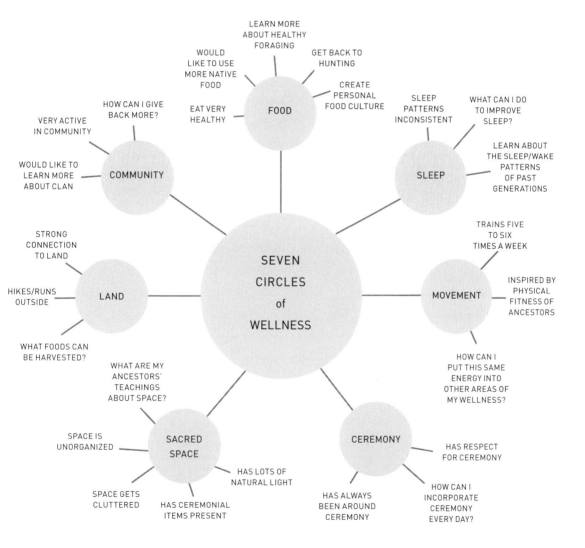

of Wellness is not a crash diet or a New Year's resolution. This is a sustainable, long-term, everlasting cycle of seeking health and wellness that you have already been participating in, whether you know it or not. Often, mainstream wellness plans are designed to throw you into an anxious, deficit mindset. They ask you to "begin" your health journey by identifying what you want to change, fix, or alter about yourself. We'd rather you begin from a place of surplus, which is much less daunting and intimidating. Ask yourself: Where am I already thriving?

Take some time to draw your own Seven Circles of Wellness, in their various sizes, as they are today. Similar to the examples under Scenarios 1 and 2, some circles will be larger, some smaller. It's up to you to decide where you are thriving and where you have opportunities to grow. Consider both conventional health-related concepts (like healthy eating) and unconventional or atypical health-related concepts (like family and community connection). Here are some examples for each circle:

- If you are a devoted grandparent or auntie, you are thriving in **community**.
- If you do not bring your phone or another device to bed with you at night, to avoid the negative aspects of blue light, and you wake up feeling refreshed, you are thriving in **sleep**.
- If you spend one day each week on an intentional social media fast, integrating silence and stillness into your day instead, you are thriving in **ceremony**.
- If you are reading recipe books and working on a nutrition plan with your doctor to emerge from your prediabetes diagnosis, you are thriving in **food**.
- If you take time to make your bed every morning, you are thriving in **sacred space**.
- If you go for regular walks with your pets or family, you are thriving in **movement**.
- If you are knowledgeable about, for instance, the Landback movement and the Indigenous history where you live, you are thriving in connection to **land**.

Now you have identified circles where you are thriving, and you have taken a moment to acknowledge your efforts and feel good about your progress. You have also identified circles that are smaller, that need more work. Rest assured that this book will leave you with ideas and inspiration for that work.

As you read, continue to reflect on your personal Seven Circles of Wellness. Use this initial drawing as a base model to create an intricate *Seven Circles mind-map* that paints a much more detailed picture of your personal vision of a balanced life. Write or draw out what you are already doing for your health, what you would like to do more of, what you would like to stop doing, which habits you would like to replace, anything you would like to learn, what questions you have, and so on. Think of people, places, sights, sounds, and senses that are related to your vision of good health. Visualization is a powerful tool. Once you see yourself in a state of balance and healing, your body, mind, and spirit will begin to move in that direction.

Returning to Reverence

By now, your mindset has shifted, your vision of what "balance" means has broadened, and you are ready to dive deeper into this book and your path to balance. We are very much with you on this journey. We may be the writers of this book, but we are not fully healed. Our Seven Circles of Wellness are always shrinking and growing; our cycles of learning, engaging, and optimizing are ongoing; and our return to balance is constantly in motion. No one is above, below, ahead, or behind anyone else on this road to living well.

But beyond balance, we hope that as a result of reading this book, you experience a return to *reverence*—a state of mind that our ancestors embodied so fully, in which all things in life are sacred, special, and worthy of care. Eliminate all thoughts of competition and comparison. This journey is yours. May it fulfill and nourish you.

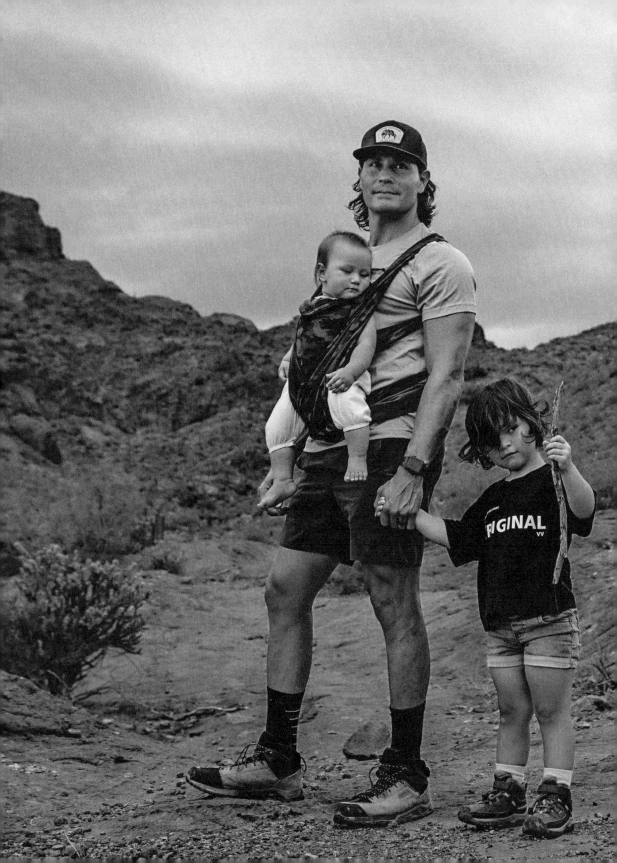

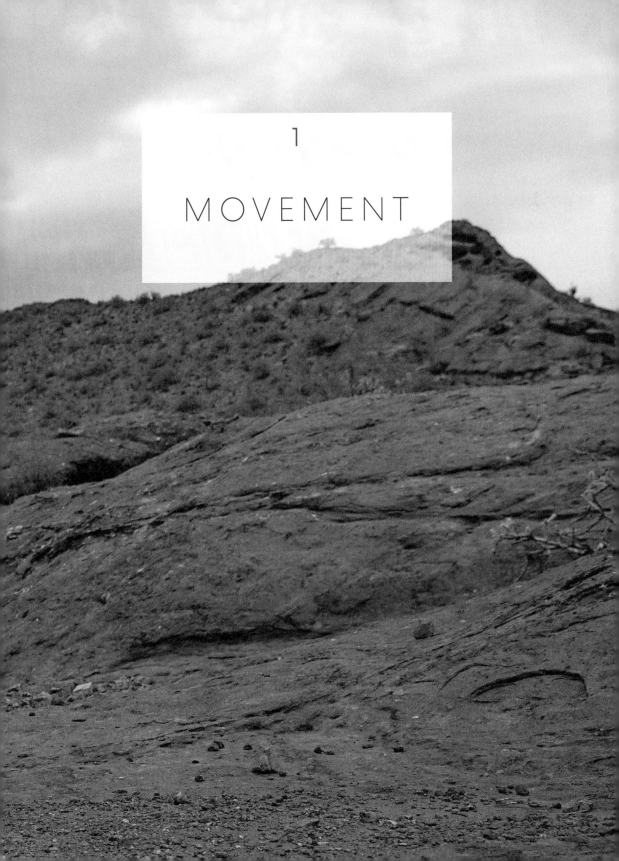

1

MOVEMENT

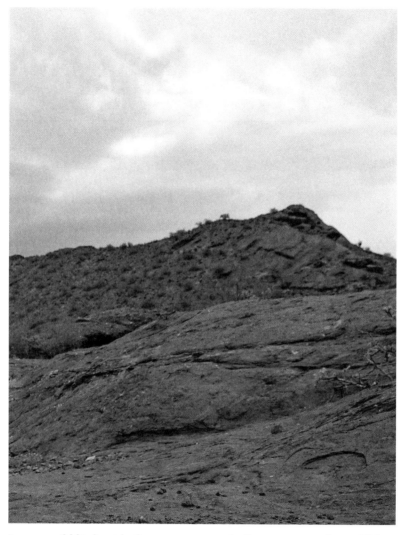

I was a wild little girl of seven . . . not wholly conscious of myself, but was more keenly alive to the fire within. It was as if I were the activity, and my hands and feet were the only experiments for my spirit to work upon.

—*Zitkala-Sa/Gertrude Simmons Bonnin (Yankton Sioux),* American Indian Stories

Previous spread: Thosh, Alo (three), and Westyn (seven months) hike by Red Mountain.

MOVEMENT IS OUR CULTURE

Nothing came between our Indigenous ancestors and their active lifestyles. Through elemental challenges, like treacherous territory or extreme weather, they moved. Through day-to-day work and play, whether harvesting food or having fun at a social dance, they moved. And during life's great transitions—those monumental human challenges that we all still face today, like aging and evolving into new stages of life—they moved. Far from the sedentary culture that most Americans are accustomed to these days, our people could not have imagined a life spent behind a desk, in front of a computer, or behind the wheel of a car. There are plenty of people now who have learned the importance of setting aside time for exercise. But that is precisely the problem—we are *setting it aside*. What we need to do is follow the Indigenous ancestral example and *integrate it*. In our experience, perhaps nothing has taught us this lesson more profoundly than our most recent rite of passage: becoming parents to our sacred little ones.

On May 2, 2017, the day we found out we were going to have a baby, it dawned on us instantly that we had no idea what we were doing. The only thing we knew for sure is that we didn't particularly relate to the advice we were reading in typical parenting magazines and books. Already committed to a wellness lifestyle rooted in ancestral teachings, we knew that we should try to extend this commitment into our parenting approach. If we could learn how our ancestors ate, exercised, and meditated, then surely we could learn how they approached pregnancy and parenting. With a baby on the way, we felt our desire to reclaim all of these aspects of Indigenous health becoming so much more urgent. Our wellness journey would now, in a very real sense, impact future generations.

We scoured the reaches of the internet for every obscure academic article we could find on ancestral Indigenous parenting. We consulted everyone in our families—aunties, uncles, moms, dads, and grandparents—who could help. We listened when they told us tips like "Don't watch violent things on TV because the baby is already taking everything in," or "Use elk teeth and dried moose meat for teething," or "Keep the infant close to you, wrapped tightly in a cradleboard—it comforts them, like the womb."

While ancestral teachings on parenting vary widely from nation to nation, this concept of using a cradleboard, or other Indigenous baby carrier, was one that came up everywhere. Inuit parents, from the far north, use the *amauti*—an animal-skin parka with a big, cozy, safe hood, allowing an infant to join arctic hunting expeditions. The Ojibwe, woodlands people, use the *dikinaagan*—a baby-carrying backpack adorned in velvet and floral beadwork. The O'odham, desert people, use the *vulkud*—an airy cradleboard, equipped with a shade made of willow, designed to protect a baby as the parents harvest food under the sun. The ubiquitous presence of Indigenous baby carriers and cradleboards, perfectly suited to the parents' environments and places of work, demonstrated the ethos of Indigenous parenting. To have a baby is to *carry* that baby, everywhere you go. An infant would not disrupt the work, life, health, or duties of a parent; instead, it would, without question, be along for the ride.

Agreeing with the philosophy of our ancestors was one thing. Of course we wanted to reject the norm of today's unforgiving society that fails to offer adequate paternity and maternity leave and that severs opportunities for new parents to bond with their babies. Certainly it sounded noble to mimic the way that our ancestors seamlessly incorporated babies and children into every aspect of daily life without conflict. On one hand, we felt confident in that we had already managed to break out of some of the constraints that modern life places on most people—we were our own bosses, who made our own hours, and this freedom played no small role in our commitment to our well lifestyle. But bringing a baby into the mix would add a whole new layer of complication. In today's nuclear-family setting, without the constant support of our *tiospaye* (extended family) and village, as would have been the case two hundred years ago, this challenge to interweave our active, healthy lifestyles with our parenting would be just that—a challenge.

Five years later, now with two daughters, well into our journey as parents, we are happy to report that with continued trial and error, some days better than others, we have pretty much figured out how to make it all work. And, we can confirm that our instinct to prioritize movement, just as our ancestors did, was spot-on. Staying active as a family has been a priceless contribution to our lives. Movement is our fun, our emotional outlet, and a shared activity that bonds us. Today, as it was for our ancestors, movement is our culture once again.

The key has been *integration*, that is, viewing movement not as an extracurricular activity, but as an essential aspect of health care, child-rearing, and total well-being. Every day, we weave movement into our schedules, no matter what else is on the agenda. We include our kids in our movement practices, rather than waiting for "me-time"; otherwise, we wouldn't get it in nearly often enough. Integrating them not only makes sense, it also instills in them good habits and confidence. They will grow up knowing that exercise is a normal and natural part of everyday of life—that people are made to move.

Our days look something like this: In between answering emails, teaching workshops online, and taking part in conference calls, we are cooking their tiny little meals to serve them on their colorful little plates, we are changing their diapers, we are negotiating screen time. Meanwhile, we keep exercise mats and open space in every room so that we can stretch or work in sets of push-ups as our kids play with their toys. Instead of using our garage for cars or storage, we have turned it into our gym so that we don't have to leave home to train and work out. They have their own mini yoga mats and tiny plastic kettlebells. They play, dance, and eat snacks as we hit the heavy bag or lift weights. We make a point of using carriers—both modern and ancestral styles—far more often than strollers, so that whether we're doing a mundane task, like grocery shopping, or enjoying a recreational outing, like hiking, they are with us and we are getting in a workout. When we take part in online meetings, we stand rather than sit, and when we are doing conference calls, we walk around, wearing headphones. Integrating movement throughout the day is possible, even in the modern world.

We do this not only for our physical fitness and preventive health care, but also because movement is our way of relieving stress, having fun, and putting our ancestral values of hard work, productivity, and inclusivity into practice. Movement has been a powerful medicine for our family, and we know that it can be for you and yours, too. By reclaiming everyday active lifestyles in our home, we are indeed carrying on the culture of our ancestors. We are also breaking down contemporary stereotypes, making a statement that being active is who we are as Native people. Just as it was normal for our ancestors' children to see Mom tanning a hide or Dad making a hunting expedition on foot, it is normal for our children to see Mom swinging a kettlebell in the garage or Dad practicing in the yard with his bow and arrow.

As we reclaim and evolve a culture of movement, we encourage a critical re-thinking of American fitness culture, and a careful application of terminology and intention. For example, we use the word "movement" instead of "fitness" because we acknowledge that "fitness" is a limited concept with intimidating connotations that fail to be inclusive. Not everyone feels welcome to fitness. "Movement," how-ever, is something that everyone can connect with and participate in. It encom-passes many modalities, including dance, breathing exercises, studio workouts, sports, swimming, food practices, parenting, ceremonies, martial arts, manual labor, outdoor activities, and so much more.

Today, Western fitness culture has skewed our view of movement in an un-healthy way. We *force* ourselves to exercise because we want to *change* our bodies. Many people hate their bodies. This mentality is harmful for our mental and emo-tional health, and it is antithetical to the healing that movement has the potential to bring to our lives. Just as our ancestors did, we prefer to tell a more complete story about movement, recognizing all that it can do for our holistic health and wellness.

The Indigenous mentality recognizes that movement is not just about recreation or physical looks. Movement is an all-encompassing medicine that can benefit us mentally, physically, spiritually, and emotionally. Movement is a celebration of life and a way of honoring and giving thanks for our bodies. It is something that we *get* to do, not something that we *have* to do. We hope that all people come to view movement as a powerful form of preventive health care, a fun part of life with family and friends, and a tremendous healing tool—not a chore or a punishment.

When we became parents, the greatest challenge of our lives to date, we discovered that we did not have to stop moving, stop living, or stop having fun. We found out that, while incredibly challenging and humbling at times, making a point of continuing to move our bodies has been emotionally fulfilling, spiritually healing, and physically rewarding. Whether the challenge that you are now facing in life is parenting, career, school, or anything else, we encourage you to *integrate* movement in your daily life, just as our people so beautifully demonstrated.

HOW MOVEMENT HEALS
⊕ Movement Medicine Wheel ⊕

SPIRITUAL
Incorporating breath, intention, and prayer with each movement practice—no matter what that movement practice is—will result in spiritual growth and a heightened connection to yourself and/or Creator.

EMOTIONAL
Different movement practices impact our emotions in different ways. Understanding this allows us to use movement as a tool to work through or with our emotions. Gratitude is a positive feeling that can be centered through movement. Giving thanks for our bodies and our ability to move turns our mindset toward healing and away from harmful thoughts like shame.

MENTAL
Movement sharpens the mind and memory. People in many Indigenous nations know that going for a run first thing in the morning or stepping outside to greet the sun with a tall posture and deep breathing helps one wake up and ignites the brain (as opposed to rolling over to scroll through a screen or reaching right away for a stimulant like caffeine).

PHYSICAL

By reintegrating movement throughout the day and consciously counteracting the sedentary lifestyle that was imposed by colonialism, we can collectively reclaim the physical durability and strength that our ancestors demonstrated. All people can take an Indigenous approach to movement, viewing it as a necessary mode of preventive health care—something that must be prioritized and integrated into our schools, homes, and workplaces once again to prevent and heal from modern diseases like heart disease, diabetes, and obesity.

Creator's Original Instructions: To Move Is to Honor Our Existence

Let my strength be like that of the mighty buffalo who rock-like withstands the prairie blizzards and fiery days. Let me be tireless on the trail so that if need be I could walk around the world.

—*Ojibwe warrior prayer, from* Ojibwe Ceremonies

Although we emphasize the importance of the inclusive, gentle side of movement, we also believe that when a person is ready and able, it is by all means a good thing to invite physical discomfort in a challenging, high-intensity movement practice. Our bodies are a gift to be honored, nourished, and cared for, and pushing our physical limits is one way of celebrating our strength. The late Albert White Hat, a Lakota knowledge keeper and educator, said that "the only possession we have, that we can claim, is our body." Training for strength and agility, then, is a way of giving the one thing that we truly have to give: our energy. A challenging movement practice is not just for a star athlete or a body builder. It is a way for everyone to prepare themselves for the moments in life when others need them.

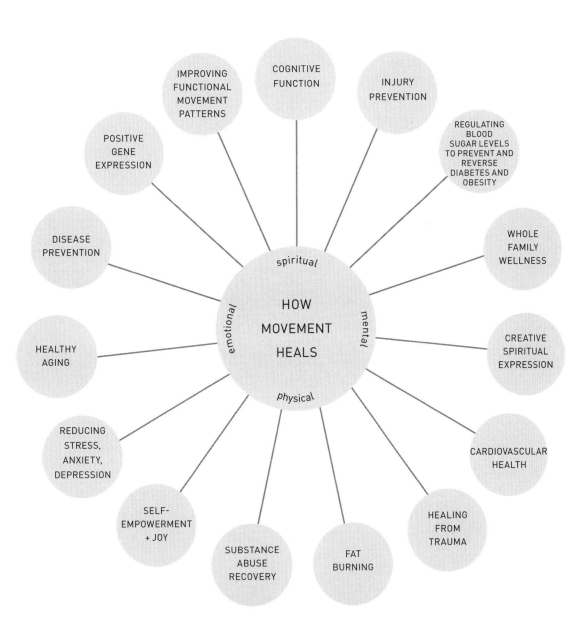

IMPROVING FUNCTIONAL MOVEMENT PATTERNS

COGNITIVE FUNCTION

INJURY PREVENTION

POSITIVE GENE EXPRESSION

REGULATING BLOOD SUGAR LEVELS TO PREVENT AND REVERSE DIABETES AND OBESITY

DISEASE PREVENTION

WHOLE FAMILY WELLNESS

spiritual

HOW MOVEMENT HEALS

emotional

mental

HEALTHY AGING

CREATIVE SPIRITUAL EXPRESSION

physical

REDUCING STRESS, ANXIETY, DEPRESSION

CARDIOVASCULAR HEALTH

SELF-EMPOWERMENT + JOY

HEALING FROM TRAUMA

SUBSTANCE ABUSE RECOVERY

FAT BURNING

"As long as you can move around, you should take care of yourself," White Hat said. "The greatest gift that you can give is time from your life."[1]

Native people from many nations have always acknowledged that movement is an essential building block for community wellness. Ohiyesa, also known as Charles Eastman, was a doctor who lived during the late nineteenth and early twentieth centuries. He wrote that during his precolonial upbringing in the north woods of Dakota territory (contemporary Minnesota), physical training was considered an act of preparation for public service. Young boys were trained to grow strong and athletic so that they could feed their families as hunters and protect their communities as warriors. Given the changing world around him, his life ended up taking a different direction from warriorhood, but he still exemplified these teachings in a new cultural context. His athletic prowess helped him to socialize and succeed as a star football player at Dartmouth College. He then earned a medical degree and served as a first-responding doctor at the massacre at Wounded Knee on the Pine Ridge Reservation, a tragedy during which the United States Army killed and injured hundreds of Lakota women, children, and elders.[2]

In Native communities, during ceremony and prayer, we always express gratitude for our bodies, for our strength, and for our abilities. The Indigenous mindset is that fitness has never been solely for aesthetics, but rather for practical application in survival, artistic expression, social gatherings, child-rearing, and peace-making. Through movement, we have formed interactions with one another, with the elements, with the plant nations, and with the animal nations, thus learning to survive and thrive in balance with the land. We grow strong, agile, and emotionally vibrant so that we can take care of one another and the world around us.

The desire to physically move is an innate human impulse, and to do so is to fulfill one of our most elemental needs as five-fingered, two-legged beings. When we are physically active, our spirits rev up and our neuronal impulses fire in all directions, causing the brain to light up. Whether it be a rhythmic, regimented, or free-form expression of movement, we thrive on movement because it is our original way of being human.

As we have mentioned, not so long ago in Indian Country, a normal lifestyle was an active lifestyle. Regular, daily tasks included building structures, processing food, hunting, maintaining fields, traveling to trade and to deliver messages, moving camp, training for warfare, swimming and running for recreation, participating in social dances and ceremonies, and so much more. Indigenous people understood that survivability was largely dependent upon the durability and fitness of each person. Everyone prioritized maintaining strength and agility so that the whole community could operate collectively and efficiently. Oral tradition says that our people often lived to be older than one hundred years, and even at that age they could walk, sit comfortably on the ground, stand up without assistance, and generally maintain a level of mobility, strength, and grit that is uncommon in elders today. In the Indigenous worldview, having a physically well body was as important as having mental clarity, regulated emotions, and a grounded spiritual state.

In the Lakota creation story, before the world and humans and all life forms existed as they do today, the *maka* (land) and *mni* (water) became united under the sky by an energy force called *takuskanskan*, which is defined as *the spiritual power that causes the movement of everything*. As humans who walk the earth today, we should remember our creation stories and continue to embody them. We may walk in a way that reflects the power of our origin stories. It is *movement* that helped to create and unite the elemental building blocks of our world. Today, by moving our bodies, we are honoring our health, the land, the water, and our spirits by flowing with *takuskanskan* rather than resisting it. To be well today, we must keep moving, keep praying, and continue to remember the spiritual power of movement that gave us land, water, energy, community, and life itself.

BUILDING FUNCTIONAL, TOTAL-BODY STRENGTH: THE SEVEN BASIC MOVEMENT PATTERNS

From sinew used as string, to tiny bones used as toothpicks, to dried organs used as water vessels, the Lakota people famously used every single part of the buffalo they hunted. Ensuring that no part of an animal's body went to waste demonstrated honor and respect for that animal's life. It was also a practical method for securing the most benefit from the effort of a hunt.

In that same vein, we encourage *using every part* of our own bodies in a movement practice. Using our whole body—from fingertips, to lungs, to the soles of our feet, to our spine—nurtures the special function of each and every part of ourselves. It honors our whole being, even those parts that we have grown to dislike or avoid. It also serves a practical purpose in developing "real-world strength" or total body fitness that makes us able to not only be strong in the gym, but also perform everyday tasks in life, like getting on all fours to scrub our floors, squatting to pick up heavy boxes, or developing upper-body strength to carry groceries. One can start the process of incorporating this dynamic, well-rounded, functional movement style by learning the *Seven Basic Movement Patterns*: push, pull, squat, lunge, hip hinge, rotate, and gait (or walk/run).

These movement patterns are taught as part of a system in the world of *functional training*. Every exercise falls within or includes at least one of these Seven Basic Movements. Notice how a toddler can easily squat to pick up a toy with perfect form. We are born to engage with these movement patterns, and we can continue to do so as long as we don't neglect the motions. No matter our age, occupation, or athletic level, we all can benefit from consciously training these fundamental patterns.

We often think about the body as a divided system, broken up into parts. Popular fitness culture today encourages this compartmentalized thinking, as commonly seen in tutorials for "eight-minute abs" or "bicep blasting." This is a body-building approach—fine for those who are focused purely on aesthetics, but

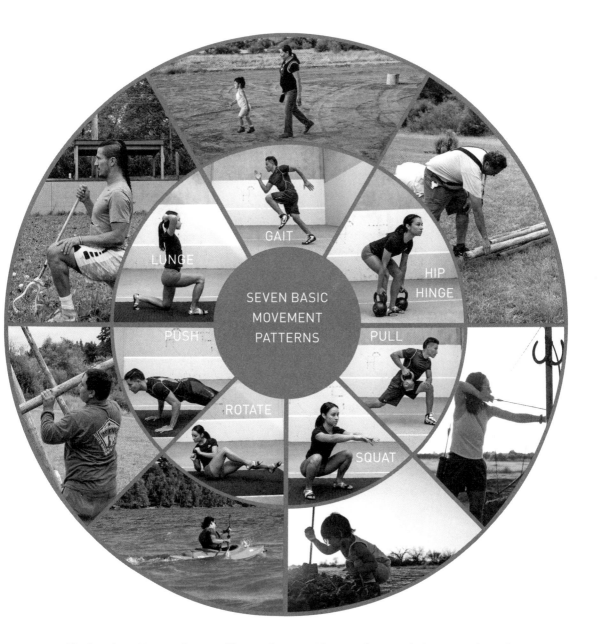

The Seven Basic Movement Patterns of functional training. The inner photos are the "training in the gym" versions, and the outer photos demonstrate "real-world" examples. Individuals pictured (starting at top center) are: Alo Collins, Jo Collins, Will Penn, Chelsey Luger, Alo Collins, Thosh Collins, Josh Cocker, and Jeremy Thompson.

less functional for overall health. In fact, the body is not neatly compartmental-ized. Like life on earth, it is all connected. For example, when you press a weight over your head, you aren't just using your arms; you are also relying on your grip, engaging your core, adjusting your hips, squeezing your legs, and balancing with your toes. The body is a single unit made up of complex, interconnected systems that work together as one. So in order to build functional, real-world strength, power, flexibility, and stamina, one should focus on training whole-body move-ment patterns rather than isolating muscle groups.

To begin incorporating the Seven Basic Movements into your fitness routine, start by performing a basic version of each pattern with your own body weight—for example, a standard squat, a standard push-up, or a standard forward lunge. Focus on executing each movement with good technique and form. Seek guid-ance and assistance from a personal trainer if you have access to one. Once you become comfortable with these basic movements, work on progressing to more complex exercises by creating dynamic, compound movements—for example, a walking lunge with an upper-body twist, or a jump-squat with weight. Learning the Seven Basic Movements will allow you to develop an arsenal of endless exer-cise ideas and workout routines. Most important, this concept will teach you to view the body as a unified, interconnected system that you can utilize holistically.

Dancing for the People: The Powwow Movement Mentality

The powwow is perhaps the most widely recognized form of Indigenous move-ment today. These community events are usually open to the public, so most people have probably seen Indigenous dancers in their beautiful, colorful rega-lia. Powwow culture perfectly captures the Indigenous movement mentality be-cause it celebrates the joy and good energy that movement can bring. Powwow is unique in that it is culturally intertribal—something that has an origin story in several nations and that today many Native people from different nations host and participate in. There are multiple categories of dance within a powwow—grass, fancy, traditional, jingle, and more. Some powwows are competitive, with

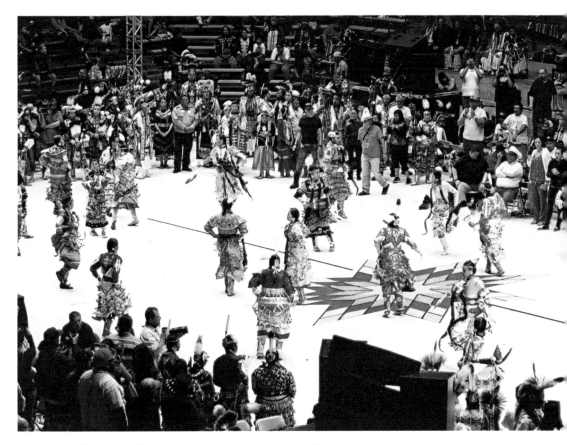

Jingle dancers from many different nations compete at the Gathering of Nations Powwow.

judges who select winners in each category to earn prize money and titles. Other powwows are "traditional" or noncompetitive.

Whether contest or not, powwows always foster artistic expression, with every dancer rooted in gratitude for their ability to move. Powwow dancers are taught that they are to dance "for the people," meaning that each step of the moccasin, shake of the bustle, or raising of the fan, along with the drum and the voices of singers, serves as a collective gift for community well-being. Dancers experience joy and empowerment while moving and seek to pass this on to anyone who watches them, especially those who are most in need of being uplifted. Powwow dancers carry compassion and empathy for the fact that not everyone can move. They recognize that since they are able, they should not take their abilities for granted. They consider it their responsibility to share, with all spectators, the joy that movement can bring.

The mentality of powwow dancers can be applied to all types of movement modalities. Often, the mainstream wellness world associates specific forms of exercise, such as yoga, with spirituality but leaves all other sports and exercises in the realm of pure physicality and competition. But in fact, every single form of movement, whether basketball, boxing, or ballet, can be viewed as much as a mindful, meditative, spiritual practice as it is a physical one. And just like powwow dancers do, the good feelings that we experience as individuals who practice movement can be shared with our loved ones who need it. Any opportunity that we have to move our bodies can be rooted in gratitude. We have the power to insert our prayers, our good intentions, and our heartfelt thoughts into each and every movement practice, no matter what it is.

When Spirit Drives the Sport: Indigenous Athletics and Activism

Sports are deeply engrained in the history and contemporary culture of Indigenous nations worldwide. To witness this, one needs only to visit a high school basketball game on any reservation in the United States, where a small-town gym will be packed with supporters of all ages; or a rugby game in New Zealand, where Maori athletes and their teammates begin each game with a *haka* (ceremonial dance); or an Indian relay on the Great Plains, where crowds cheer on bareback riders in traditional horse races. In Native Country, sport is more than just a game. It is a spiritual pursuit. It is familial pride. It is an ancient calling that runs through centuries of kin and clans. Athletes learn to view their talent not just as a way to gain personal glory, but as a gift to be shared with their community. In Indigenous traditions, sport is sacred. The duty of a star athlete is not to win, but to bring a smile to an elder's face.

Indigenous sports aren't exactly as they were in ancestral times, of course. Plains Cree teenagers once trained for warfare on horseback, but now they are

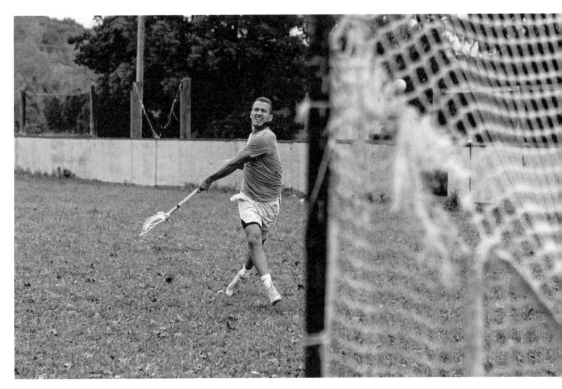

Jeremy Thompson (Onondaga), a professional lacrosse player, incorporates his spiritual values while playing the sport that his ancestors created and gifted to the world.

strapping on their hockey skates. Hopi teens once ran from village to village as messengers, but now they are state champions in high school cross-country running.[3] As different as the contexts may be, the spirit has remained. Lakota basketball players approach their game with the same fervor that was historically reserved for buffalo hunting.

All successful Native athletes share one winning trait: they play the game with their cultural values at their core. They go out there to represent their communities, their nation, and their ancestors. While not exclusively driven by competition, the Indigenous mentality happens to lead to success. We've seen this throughout history and today. The legendary Jim Thorpe (Sac and Fox) is a prime example. In 1912, he won Olympic gold in the decathlon and pentathlon. Today, he is universally recognized as one of the greatest athletes of all time.[4]

In some cases, competitive sports are a chance to bolster Indigenous nationhood in a very real political sense. Haudenosaunee lacrosse players, whose ancestors invented the sport, continue to remind us that they are playing more than just a game. The 2010 Iroquois Nationals team was famously denied a shot at a world championship when the host country, Britain, did not allow them to enter British borders using their Haudenosaunee passports, asking them instead to use US or Canadian identification. The team then refused to go, stating that they would represent themselves as the Iroquois Nationals from the Haudenosaunee Confederacy or they would not represent themselves at all.[5] The issue came up again in 2022 when the Haudenosaunee were not recognized as a sovereign nation by World Lacrosse and thus were denied a spot in the World Games. Ireland's team then gave up their spot for the Iroquois Nationals, acknowledging that lacrosse would not exist were it not for the Iroquois people gifting it to the world.[6]

Indigenous runners today are showing the world how to fuse sport with social justice. In 2019, Jordan Marie Brings Three White Horses Daniel (Lakota and Diné) started running high-profile marathons with a red handprint painted across her face to raise awareness of the overlooked crisis of Native American women, girls, and LGBTQ people going missing and/or dying by homicide at higher rates than women of any other ethnicity. Meanwhile, these crimes go largely unresolved because of jurisdictional complexities and racism in the justice system. Daniel chose the bold visual of the red handprint because it is impossible to ignore, and it makes a statement—Native women will not be silenced any longer.[7] She continues to advocate for this cause through her nonprofit organization Rising Hearts.[8]

The Native American approach to basketball helped to create the greatest basketball team of all time: the Chicago Bulls of the 1990s, led by coach Phil Jackson to six NBA championships. In the book *Sacred Hoops: Spiritual Lessons of a Hardwood Warrior*, he and Hugh Delehanty write about how Lakota philosophy and spirituality greatly influenced Jackson's coaching strategy. He took note of the impressive level of teamwork and deeply engrained spiritual commitment that young players on the Pine Ridge Reservation incorporated into their game. He adapted this notion that the basketball season was not just a competition, but a spiritual quest for all players. He taught the likes of Michael Jordan, Scottie Pippen, and Dennis Rodman how to emulate this. In short, the Chicago Bulls, in their heyday, may never have been the team they were if not for guidance from the Lakota worldview.[9]

BECOMING SELF-ACTUALIZED
THROUGH MOVEMENT
THOSH

My first experience seriously training one of the movement patterns was with gait—or running. Then, I had never heard of functional training, or the seven basic movements—I was simply participating in the spiritual life of my community. When I was nine, along with my dad and brothers, I was initiated into a men's circle whose members participated in a ceremony that required young men to run from one sacred site to another—all the while praying for a cause. Running has always been an integral aspect of an Indigenous way of life, serving as a means of communication between villages, as a sport for fun, and as a tool for spiritual growth. Today, ceremonial or spiritual runs still happen throughout the various O'odham communities for various purposes.

When I was a kid I heard elders speak at community gatherings about how our people were excellent runners and used to run all the way to the ocean to trade goods with the people who lived near there. Elders always talked about how things were done in the "old days." I remember thinking how hard our ancestors' lives sounded. I didn't want to take time away from playing Nintendo to have to run all the way to the ocean!

But sure enough, the time did come for me to run. And sure enough, it was difficult—the biggest challenge I would face as a kid, but also the most character-building. First, for four days we could drink only water and eat only fruit and *kui cu'i* (mesquite flour). We weren't allowed to have any processed, sweet, or savory foods or drinks—not even meat, because our ancestors always viewed meat as a luxury. To go without comforting food was a way to truly sacrifice. And to sacrifice one's comfort for a cause, our people teach, is how one gives oneself for others.

Fasting for health has become a trend today, but our people have always done it. It helped us to prepare our minds and bodies for the seventeen-mile initiation run from S-ve:g Do'ag (Red Mountain) to the central part of the reservation where everyone lived. The act of giving up something so vital was one of the most powerful ways for us young ones to learn humility, and to ensure that the greater purpose of the run was met.

The purpose of this particular running ceremony was to honor our ancestors whose remains had been uncovered at a construction site near Phoenix. As commercial and private development has covered O'odham territory, volumes of Indigenous material culture and remains continue to be found. The Native American Graves Protection and Repatriation Act of 1990 requires human remains and sacred objects to be treated with dignity and respect and to be returned to the lineal descendants. Leaders in our community developed a ceremony to address this, because they felt it necessary to rebury these people and their belongings in a respectful way at a place where they would never be disturbed again. Running plays a vital role in this ceremony to honor our ancestors. Out of respect for the cultural integrity of the ceremony, I can share only so much about these gatherings. But I share what little I do because I believe these stories exemplify how movement is not only physical, but also spiritual and very much about community and connection to the land.

I learned that we emit a kind of spiritual energy when we have a thought in mind that is accompanied with emotion and physical exertion. When we run for a purpose, the energy we give becomes part of the collective consciousness aimed toward healing our people or bringing attention to a social issue. Through this spiritual running process, we can elevate our own consciousness to receive new understandings and a more well-rounded outlook that will help us on our life journey. At our ceremonial runs, a community leader would give a speech reminding us what we were running for. We were told that it was not a race, nor was it for show, but it was for the spiritual health of the people. We were encouraged to pray for ourselves and for our families and our communities as we ran. The leader reminded us to think good thoughts and to pray for the people who lived in the communities through which we were running. One man once said as we ran through villages, we were like a boat going through calm water, leaving a ripple behind. We had to focus on leaving behind good thoughts and energy.

Hearing concepts like this over the years taught me that running is more than just mastering the technicalities of breath, foot strike, and stride. It goes beyond the pursuit to improve cardiovascular fitness or achieve a personal feat of strength. Deeper spiritual teachings about running taught me that our personal health is in many ways a reflection of the collective health of the people. When we are strong as nations, it is because we are carried by ancestral knowledge, practices, and a community of people who are oriented toward future generations.

A few years after becoming a spiritual runner, I started playing basketball with the Salt River Warriors, a team led by Robert Johnston (Creek and Choctaw), a coach, wellness advocate, and mentor who continues to influence and change the lives of many Native youth. In his style of coaching, he integrated Indigenous teachings of kinship, honor, love, leadership, and commitment. Those teachings helped strengthen my sense of belonging and confidence, which boosted my leadership skills and made my fire strong. This was an especially important perspective to hear as a Native kid in the 1980s who easily could have been influenced by the drugs and alcohol that were starting to become prevalent on my reservation and in the surrounding city at that time.

Later, I applied the same mentality to breakdancing—an artistic form of movement that was a positive creative outlet that also informed my personal movement culture. The first time I saw breakdancing was at a teen dance held at the Salt River multipurpose building. Me and my good friends We:Whum, Quetzal, Breeze, Alex, and Angelo were instantly hooked and started immersing ourselves in the local underground hip hop culture, learning how to break through VHS tapes like

Beat Street. Soon we became a real b-boy crew who started to travel and compete. Our dance style organically evolved beyond the traditional confines of what was considered breakdancing and was more "street dance." We were known for our creativity and made our mark on the international street dance scene.

In retrospect, I realize that as young Native men, we still carried in us the desire to rhythmically move our bodies and express ourselves like our ancestors had before us. We were just doing it differently because our peoples' original dancing practices had been interrupted by colonialism.

The good feelings we got while dancing provided a sense of fulfillment similar to what we experienced during spiritual runs, but the dynamism of breakdancing allowed me to develop a new kind of appreciation for physical movement. In my early twenties, I moved to California and was introduced to even more modalities of movement, such as yoga, capoeira, mixed martial arts, and functional fitness. I was attracted to these styles of movement because of their dynamic athleticism and philosophies about spirituality and community. Each of these modes was practical in a health-care sense but also was an outlet of expression and a way for me to let go of some of the pain and stress I'd been carrying around—pain that for a long time I couldn't pinpoint but that led me to give in to the peer pressures of alcohol and substance abuse.

I made it to age twenty-one without drinking alcohol and was staunchly against it because of my upbringing. But when I started, I began to ask myself why I was now allowing it into my life. Every time I drank or took drugs I knew it was not a good way of life for me. The voices of my parents and elders in my community rang in my head, cautioning me against it as I went on party rages with friends in the city. Sometimes my parents and elders would even show up in my dreams and scold me. But I always justified it and continued to reassure myself that one day I'd quit—just not now because I was having too much fun.

As I continued to drink more, I no longer had the desire to dance, and I could feel my fire start to dim. I eventually lost my job, and I was ashamed of myself for letting that happen. For a year I couch-surfed around LA and made occasional trips home and other places to do photography work. Even though I had no home in LA, I still kept going back because I thought my social life was missing out.

I began to become worried about the direction I was headed. And then Robert, my old basketball coach, began to invite me to come back to the Native Wellness Institute's healing and wellness gatherings that I used to attend as a youth. Around 2010–2011 I started returning to their gatherings where I listened to speakers and took part in talking circles. It became clearer than ever how my family, community, and I have been affected by historic intergenerational trauma.

While growing up on the rez I'd always heard people address how our hardships were due to our loss of land and culture, but newer findings about cultural trauma opened my eyes to a new level of understanding. I started learning about how the Native wellness community was beginning to change the way they addressed health disparities and promote a narrative about healing through our cultural lifeways. It dawned on me how experiencing premature deaths of friends and family due to a high prevalence of health disparities on the reservation had resulted in multilayered and complex grief accumulating within me. I was full of unaddressed grief and anger after the tragic deaths of my brother Steven and sister Dovey. I knew I needed to make lifestyle changes to prevent myself from going down a path of suffering and addiction.

I knew I had the tools to heal because I was raised with them, but I needed to muster up enough strength to apply them as an adult. In 2011 I moved back to the rez to be close to family and community again. And finally in 2013, I got out of an unhealthy relationship and quit using alcohol and other substances. Around that time I picked up Transcendental Meditation through the Native Wellness Institute. It was time to focus and start thinking about my future.

I got myself a small bachelor pad and was intent on living a clutter-free and minimal lifestyle. I immersed myself into learning traditional O'odham songs and sang at community events. I started to change the way I was eating. I found myself back on the land, hiking, hunting, and learning about desert plants alongside my brother Amson. I also started doing what I call Earth Gym, where I take my training out on the land for a different fitness experience. I used anything, from rocks to logs, to lift and used cliffs and ledges to do pull-ups. I was inspired by the Indigenous games taught by the late Charles Tailfeathers at Native Wellness Institute summer youth camps.

Charlie was a Cree/Blackfeet elder from Rocky Boy, Montana, living on the Warm Springs Reservation in Oregon with his wife, Nancy, and their grandchildren. He was also a board member and facilitator of the Native Wellness Institute. He taught various Indigenous games that he had participated in when he was growing up. He always emphasized that the games were a test of agility, speed, strength, and endurance. Some of them required players to pick a stone and run an uphill course while carrying water in their mouths. This left them with only nasal breathing, for an added challenge to their endurance. Charlie told stories of how people considered it good medicine to come out to watch these games.

When I showed him some of the Earth Gym videos that Chelsey and I made, he endorsed it and encouraged us to share Earth Gym with youth. What I love about Earth Gym is the escape from the indoor mainstream fitness culture. I love being out on the land, feeling the elements and breathing the fresh air. On the land, there are no even surfaces or soft handles for our convenience; there is only the land and its tough love to help us develop grit, connection, and real-world strength.

Since I was no longer going out to drink several times a week, I was sleeping better and noticed a positive change in my mood and outlook. I had more energy and mental drive to start training at the Salt River Fitness Center, where I spent the next eight years being trained by Coach Dion Begay, who is originally from the Navajo Nation. Dion holds several degrees in exercise science and works as a trainer at Salt River's Diabetes Prevention Department. Functional fitness became my new go-to modality of movement. After quitting alcohol and changing my lifestyle, I needed a hybrid way to build my fire back up, and flinging kettlebells, slamming med balls, kicking heavy bags, and sprinting really ignited a different kind of spirit power in me. It was the most fun and engaging way to keep my mind sharp, body strong, and emotions balanced for the kind of life I wanted to live—doing things on the land and partaking in community.

During my workouts I'd recall the years of running when elders would say to us,

"Pray for the people when you run!" It made sense to me that this teaching could be applied to modern fitness culture in Native communities whose goals were disease prevention. Oftentimes while working out I felt as if I was contributing to this collective idea where Native people are consciously Indigenizing modern fitness to reclaim our health and identity. I didn't know it at the time, but I was applying the Seven Circles of Wellness as a lifestyle intervention. With a clearer vision of my place in the community, I had a new appreciation for what the rez had offered, and I found myself getting involved in community affairs. After a while, I felt proud of how quickly I had been able to pull myself back together. I had a positive vision of myself in the future being successful, financially stable, healthy, and busy.

Ever since then, movement has been my medicine. I've made it a part of my *himdag*, my way of life. That is the mindset that I've adopted, and it has helped me to keep on a path where movement is as essential to life as eating. By exemplifying this, I hope to make this the norm once again for our daughters, and to inspire all people to ground themselves and heal through movement.

MOVEMENT FOR LEARNING

Western culture often divides and compartmentalizes. It designates school and work as mental practices, while physical fitness is an entirely separate pursuit. But the brain and body work together as one. When we exercise the muscles of the mind and body together, we can cultivate their mutual effectiveness. Integrating movement in learning can help us work faster and smarter, meanwhile making the learning process more interactive and enjoyable. Science has overwhelmingly agreed with ancestral knowledge that movement ignites and develops the brain. By promoting the production of brain-derived neurotropic factor (BDNF), movement improves cognitive function, and people who regularly move demonstrate better concentration, sharpness, and memory.[10]

The medicine man Frank Fools Crow always took time to sit on the ground for mindful breathing exercises before engaging in his healing work.[11] President Barack Obama did a half hour of cardio every day before leading the United States. Great leaders and teachers know that we must fuse mental and physical tasks. Many of us cite our busy schedules as the reason for not having time to exercise, not realizing that when we move our bodies, even for a few minutes each day, our mind works better, and we can get more done in the time that we do have. Movement takes time and energy, but it also creates time and energy.

After we offered this perspective during one of our workshops, a law school student took our advice and shared her results with us a few months later. She said that she started integrating one hour of movement into her daily study schedule, no longer viewing it as a break, but as part of the process. This shift in mindset made all the difference for her. It allowed her to be consistently physically active without feeling guilty about it. She experienced an improvement in academic performance and mental clarity and found that moving regularly helped her to study more energetically and efficiently.

Moving With and Through Our Emotions

Science agrees with the ancestral understanding that movement lifts our spirits. By triggering "feel-good" neurotransmitters and hormones, like serotonin, dopamine, and endorphins, movement makes us feel happy and at ease.[12] In our own movement practices, where we include everything from breakdancing to mixed martial arts to ceremonial runs, we have observed that different types of movement modalities elicit different emotional responses. Thus, we have the power to enhance or quell various feelings by strategically using a corresponding movement. For example, hitting a heavy bag in a boxing class can be a healthy outlet for releasing anger or aggression, while stretching with deep breaths can create feelings of contentedness and calm.

We encourage everyone to experiment and find out what type of emotion you experience in response to different movements. These won't be the same for everyone. Through trial and error, you can find out which movements help you to relieve stress, to bring peace, or to release anger.

Once your emotional responses to movement become clear, you can consciously incorporate movement into your routine for mental health and healing. The goal is not to neglect or avoid emotions and feelings, but rather to partner with them in a meaningful way. No one should expect themselves to feel positive all the time, but everyone can empower themselves by honing this inherent ability to literally and figuratively move in and out of certain mental or emotional states.

We do not suggest that movement should replace other forms of behavioral health care. In fact, we strongly encourage counseling, therapy, talking circles, ceremonies, or any other approach that works for you. In an ideal world, all people would be comfortable seeking professional help for mental health and would have access to many forms of therapy. But we are forced to reckon with the reality that many people do not have access to these resources, so it is worth exploring the idea of movement as a personal healing outlet, especially in cases when few other tools are available. In this context, movement can be viewed as a form of social justice, offering much-needed support to people and communities who face historical and intergenerational trauma, while also experiencing a lack of access to health insurance and other resources.

MOVEMENT AS ARTISTIC EXPRESSION, ART, AND ORAL TRADITION

If you ever sit down to visit with a Native grandpa, auntie, or other storyteller, you will quickly see that their stories cannot be told without movement. The arms and hands swoop out and around, mimicking birds or deer or gusts of wind. The head and neck follow the path of the animals or vehicles being described. The ponytail or braid swooshes from side to side from underneath a cowboy hat or trucker cap. And of course, the head is thrown back in laughter at some point or another. Stories are more than just conversation for Indigenous communities. They carry teachings, virtues, ceremonial instructions, history, and the essence of our very distinct sense of humor.

In many Native communities, certain stories are so important that they are told only during specific times of the year, by people who were appointed to tell them, because a story told at the wrong time or in the wrong way might bring bad medicine. So people look forward to winter storytellings, for example, in the same way that a person from another culture would look forward to Christmas. These gatherings are an opportunity for the community to hear the storyteller speak the Indigenous language fluently, for the people to be reminded of the nation's origin, and for everyone to remember the many lessons and morals of life that are to be followed—so as not to run into the same trouble as the characters in the story.

Movement and grand theatrics of the body are deeply woven into these oral traditions. The storyteller is always a person who can use not just their words but also their body to express the story in all of its splendor. Using the body, hands, and gestures to "talk story" is something that is also held dear in many other cultures around the world. We encourage everyone to recognize movement as so much more than just exercise. It is a means of artistic expression and education. When we use our bodies to tell the same stories that our people have been telling for thousands of years, we come to realize that movement holds invaluable knowledge of history.

Recent studies have shown the power of movement when used in conjunction with storytelling. Gestures are a form of extraverbal communication that often carry a message more directly to a listener's subconscious than the words themselves, telling the parts of the story for which there are no words. A story told or a lesson taught with gesture improves memory, comprehension, and retention in listeners or viewers.[13] Keep this in mind as you teach and communicate in your own life. It is technically effective to be physically expressive. So do not suppress your urge to "talk" with your hands and body. And as you learn new things, seek out lessons and teachers who are physically expressive. Lean in to your tendency to use movement in all types of communication, whether you are singing a song with your child or giving a presentation at work.

Another often unrecognized form of movement is visual art. Gathering clay for pottery and sculpture; tanning, sewing, and painting massive buffalo, elk, or moose hides for regalia and tipis; carving larger-than-life trees for totems; whittling animal bones or mining turquoise for jewelry—all of these art forms, and many other styles of art from around the globe, require immense physical strength, durability, and dedication. They often demand that the artist spend time outdoors, on the land, no matter the discomforts that weather, wind, and water may bring. Visual artists today might consider the idea of intentionally embracing the physically demanding aspects of their craft, acknowledging it as their workout. Though not a typical sport or fitness pursuit, this certainly is a movement practice.

MOVING OUTDOORS: EARTH GYM

Americans today spend approximately 90 percent of their time indoors—a far cry from the outdoor-oriented lifestyles of our ancestors.[14] With poor indoor air quality and a lack of spirit-boosting sunshine, it's no wonder that today, we experience so many ailments and mood disorders that our ancestors often did not experience. One of the best ways to enhance an existing movement practice, to boost mood, and to improve overall health is to utilize what we call the Earth Gym. Let the land be your equipment and the forest, mountain, yard, or city park your facility. In the Earth Gym, exercise becomes a full sensory experience—the fresh air, challenge of the elements, and openness of the sky above all add richness to the process.

In 1921, Dr. Charles Eastman predicted the future. He had witnessed the beginning stages of America's increasingly indoor, sedentary culture and knew even then that too much sitting and time spent indoors would cause widespread health problems. He predicted that one day, schools, parents, and teachers would recognize the health benefits of moving and learning outdoors.[15]

Exactly one hundred years later in 2021, during the coronavirus pandemic, outdoor-oriented private schools began to see a tenfold increase in demand for enrollment, and an increasing number of conventional schools began to experiment with outdoor classrooms for at least part of the day.[16] Eastman had been right. It's good for kids, and everyone, to get outside. It doesn't distract or hinder learning; it boosts it.[17] "The gymnasium is not the best place to develop your muscles," Eastman wrote. "[T]he formative age should season [your] muscles in the sun, in the fresh air, in the spring water coming down from the mountain . . . that is where you get your nerve tonic."[18]

There are many ways to approach the Earth Gym. You can try strength training and functional fitness on the land, using a heavy rock or log to lift as your weight instead of conventional equipment in a gym, like dumbbells or machines. You can try water-based workouts, like kayaking, surfing, or swimming. You can simply take a walk, jog, or hike outside, rather than using a treadmill. You can even bring your studio workouts, like yoga or Pilates, to the outdoors, whether in your backyard, on your rooftop, or in a city park. Of course, real-world tasks like playing with your children, cleaning up your yard, or working in your garden count too. If you are outside and moving your body, this is Earth Gym.

Earth Gym is one of the foundational, core concepts that we began to teach and incorporate when we first launched Well For Culture. It has been exciting to see this movement grow—not just from within the Indigenous community, but among all types of people in the functional movement scene and beyond. When all gyms closed at the beginning of the coronavirus pandemic in 2020, a huge surge in learning how to exercise outdoors occurred. It proved what we have always said: gyms and equipment are great, but we shouldn't completely rely on them. All one truly needs is their body weight and a small area of space to move.

Utilizing the Earth Gym can also be a social justice statement. Elite gyms, private clubs, and expensive studios in wealthy neighborhoods need not be considered the top tier or the best form of exercise. We can train for strength, agility, and flexibility by using our bodies and the land. Truly, there is no greater venue than our earth.

MOVEMENT: AN ANTIDOTE TO ADDICTION
CHELSEY

Innate athleticism or physical strength is not a prerequisite or requirement for a solid, sustainable movement practice. What we really need lies in the spirit: a sense of will and self-determination that allows us to feel deserving of prioritizing health. It took me a long time to get to the point where this finally clicked for me. But when it did, life got a lot easier, and many things started falling into place. My hope is that young people reading this can learn from my story and spare themselves some of the trouble and heartache that I went through.

It was summer and I was sixteen. I wore beaded hemp necklaces, my lips and eyebrows were pierced, and my long dark hair was dyed with bright blue streaks. It wasn't the typical look for a girl at a small-town rodeo, but by then I was used to not fitting in. Shuffling back and forth between my mom and stepdad's house in a big college town to my dad's on a rural reservation, I constantly heard racist remarks from my white friends and challenges of "realness" from my Native friends. It wasn't cool then to be Indigenous, to be different, or to be socially conscious, and I was all of those things. But I was also just a teenager who wanted to be liked. So I learned to drink Coors Light and to down shots of cheap vodka. That helped me fit in anywhere in North Dakota, where the influence of alcohol did not discriminate.

My cousin rode in the saddle bronc contest that day, so I stuck around with him to celebrate. I showed a fake ID to get a wristband for unlimited plastic cups of beer. One minute I was two-stepping to a country song, and the next, I was blinded by a pair of flashlights shining in my face. The cops took me straight to jail.

My dad drove ninety-six miles to pick me up early the next morning. It was a

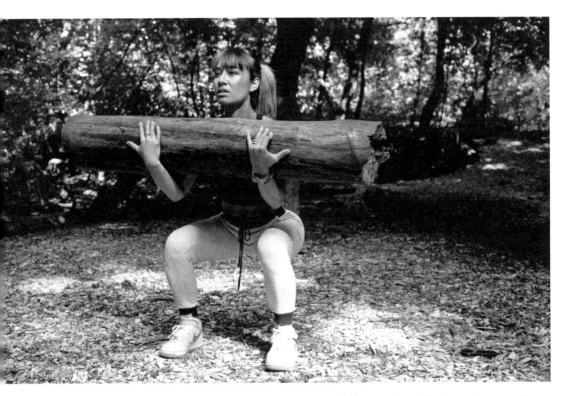

If you can find an Earth Gym in New York City, you can find one anywhere. Chelsey squats, using a log as her weight, in Prospect Park.

silent, long ride home. I kept my face pointed toward the car window in hopes my breath didn't smell as bad as it tasted. I wanted to throw up—both from dehydration and from embarrassment. I wish I could say that the feeling of shame and fear that I experienced was a big life lesson that somehow sparked a change in me, but instead, it was just the beginning of a string of incidents over years spent partying hard and facing all kinds of music: blackouts, fights, emotional outbursts, running from the cops, sneaking out, shallow friendships, breaking curfew, missing class, then waiting for my hangover to end so I could do it all again.

Back at my mom and stepdad's house, with my white friends, the rebellious behavior continued. Thankfully, the structure of my strict household was enough to keep me focused on academics, and I got into Dartmouth. There, I adored my classes in history and Native American studies, I held down three jobs, and I found good friends from all over the world. Yet my grades kept slipping and I could never reach my full potential because I was too caught up in partying. I felt like I was always falling behind, covering my own tracks, or barely skimming by. At some point, about halfway through college, I realized just how much drinking was holding me back, and I started to make a change.

My first big realization was that I had a responsibility to better represent my family and community who so lovingly raised me, because I truly was at college because of their sacrifices. I buckled down to schoolwork and slowed down on nightlife. I began regrounding myself in the teachings and values that I had learned in the Sun Dance and sweat lodge ceremonies I grew up attending with my dad. None of my spiritual leaders drank alcohol. In fact, they very profoundly demonstrated the beauty of life without it. After a holiday break, I returned to campus with two important items from home: a braid of sweetgrass to smudge with, and an eagle plume tied to a porcupine-quilled medicine wheel—something that was gifted to me in my naming ceremony when I was a little girl. I always had a cultural toolbox to guide me. It was up to me to embrace those tools.

The next thing I realized was that if I were ever going to be healthier, I needed to be honest with myself about where I was out of balance. I evaluated my life through the lens of the medicine wheel. Mentally, I was focused on rigorous academics. Spiritually, I was rooted. Emotionally, I had a good support system. But physically—well, my physical health was the piece that I had been neglecting. I worked up the courage to start going to the gym—a place I was not then comfortable or familiar with. After a while, I developed a love for weight training, and I tried studio classes like yoga and modern dance. For the first time since childhood, I felt the unhindered, joyous rush of endorphins that movement could bring.

I moved to New York City after college, where my wellness journey continued with its ups and downs. Healing is very much a nonlinear process. During those years, like most young people, I felt a lot of pressure to figure out who I was, what I wanted to be, and how I could ultimately contribute to the world around me in a meaningful way. It was hard to stay focused on grad school when I kept hearing bad news from home. I won't go into detail—I choose to keep the stories of my relatives private—but I will say that alcohol- and drug-related death and devastation continued to befall my family. It was heartbreaking.

I felt helpless, until the final and perhaps most important realization came to me. I might not become the tribal attorney who argues a landmark case in federal court, or the entrepreneur who makes a million dollars by age thirty, but I could make a real, tangible difference in my family and community by demonstrating a new normal. I could be the grandchild, the sister, the cousin, and one day even the mom who lives a good, healthy, fun, and exciting life with no substances necessary. I knew that my relatives who did not survive their traumas would want me to walk a less painful path than the one they endured. My choice to stop drinking and to focus instead on healthy living was, and still is, an act of solidarity with those who have suffered from addiction.

After I quit for good, an immense weight was lifted off my shoulders, and even though I faced whispery judgment and side-eyes from the NYC crowd who thought it odd to be sober, I felt confident and clear headed. Without drinks and hangovers, I had a lot more time on my hands, so I leaned in to my fitness interests more than ever before. I started taking classes all over Manhattan. Boxing, crossfit, Pilates, Muay Thai, ballet, animal flow, and aerial yoga would be my new modes of recreation. Taking these classes helped me to meet new people, showed me parts of the city I hadn't yet seen, and gave me a new sense of community. In this way, movement became a very practical tool that showed me I could have fun and find plenty to do outside of the status quo social scene.

I went through a few early hiccups with my relationship to movement. Body insecurities and pressure from social media left me too focused on sculpting this or trimming that. But eventually, as I continued to connect the dots between my cultural teachings and my wellness practice, my movement mentality shifted toward a much safer place. I began to accept myself in all of my imperfections, to honor and give thanks for my body rather than to nitpick it, and to know movement as my temple, my therapist, my friend, my teacher, and my art.

Right around that time, I met Thosh. He just so happened to be on the same path of sobriety, wellness, and cultural revitalization that I was on—and so we became fast friends. The first time we hung out I felt safe to talk openly with him about the very real problems we saw in our respective homelands. In between these deep conversations, we also window shopped, tried restaurants, and laughed so hard we cried. He impressed me with his duality as both a sharply dressed gentleman and a goofball with a very rez sense of humor. We put our minds together and decided then and there that we would join forces to make something of our shared passion for Indigenous wellness. We created Well For Culture, and the rest is history.

Now, a decade sober and married with two kids, I can honestly say that I have more energy, more confidence, and more of a drive for life than I ever experienced in my youth. Our career and shared passion grew organically and authentically out of our love for our communities and the intersection of our personal healing journeys. I never forget to reflect on the other paths I could have gone down. Mine is not a story of hitting "rock bottom," but I am not above the idea that it could have been. Understanding this, I approach each day with a visceral sensation of gratitude—a knowing that the strength and healing power of my Indigenous culture anchored me and outweighed the pull of the postcolonial traumas and hardships that nearly took control.

My biggest goal now is to help my daughters foster a relationship to movement that is healing, not harmful. I am making a conscious effort to pass on an important lesson that my mom always demonstrated. She raised me and my sisters in a way that eased the burden of society's fixation on image. Instead of criticizing or commenting on our looks, she praised us when we were respectful, brave, polite, or funny. She commended us for being close to our grandmothers, or for doing good work in school. Because she showed us, time and time again, that our value had nothing to do with our appearance, and because she never compared us to each other, I have been able to ultimately emerge from insecurities imposed upon me by the image-focused lens of the dominant culture.

I want the rising generation of youth to know that we are not our trauma, and we are not beholden to a fate of hardship, even if it has been the experience in our lineage. And we are not, by any means, our stereotypes. When you, your family, and your community have been through a struggle, it does not make you broken; it makes you resilient.

Today, every time I move, I set an intention for my practice, whether it be weights, stretching, or a walk outside. I recite words of gratitude quietly in my head. I am grateful for my body, and I am willing to sacrifice my own comfort so that I can become stronger in service of others. I move to honor and grow through the interaction of my mind, my spirit, and my physical self. I am grateful to all of the powerful women who came before me, who carried generations in their wombs and allowed me to do the same. I am grateful for the opportunity to heal, to nurture, and to pray through movement. After I say these words, I express them by moving.

TAKE ACTION: HOW TO INDIGENIZE YOUR MOVEMENT PRACTICE

Learn

- View movement as an all-encompassing, mental-physical-spiritual-emotional medicine that is critical for health care and overall well-being.
- Approach your personal movement practice as an opportunity to honor and celebrate the body, not as punishment or self-shame.
- Through experimentation and trial and error, figure out what type of movement you enjoy. Try classes online, at a studio, or at your local wellness center. Read about different types of movement in blogs, books, and magazines to decide what you want to try. Use social media as a tool for positive inspiration and learning.
- Consult with a physician, trainer, or other expert who can help you to determine exercises that are safe for and accessible to you.

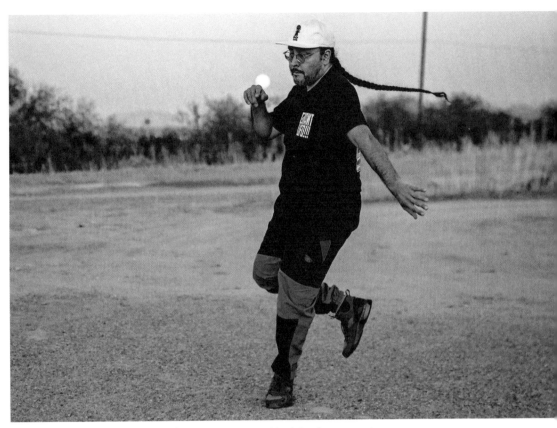

We:whum Fulwilder competes in street dance competitions worldwide but loves to practice at home on the rez.

- Learn the Seven Basic Movement Patterns for functional training. These are the basic building blocks for countless exercise combinations.
- Create and identify spaces where you can move that are affordable, safe, and accessible. This could be in your home, an outdoor area, a gym, or anywhere else that you can think of.
- In order to prevent injury, learn about the importance of warming up before strenuous exercise. Try dynamic stretches, breathing exercises, walking, and other light movements that can ease your body into exercise.

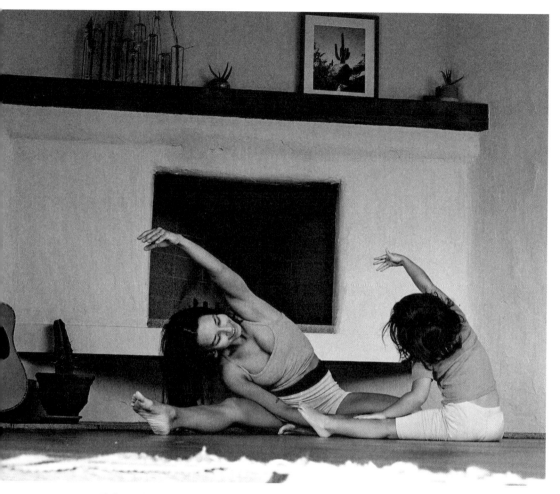

Chelsey and Alo (age three) stretch together.

- Choose a specific time of day and/or day of the week as your designated daily movement time, and aim to keep that time prioritized in your schedule. Know that you can additionally do small movements throughout the day.
- Identify any barriers that you are experiencing that prevent you from moving or that make movement seem difficult. Acknowledge the validity of these barriers, but also set an intention to overcome them.

Engage

- Using a mind-map or other brainstorming technique, design your personal movement culture—list all the reasons that movement is important in your life, all of the ways that movement can heal, and all of the people who you would like to join or support you in your movement practice.

- Recruit a support system of friends and family who are willing to move with you. Use the approach of encouragement and mutual positive reinforcement rather than shaming or teasing. Start having conversations with your network about the ways that you can work together and support one another in a consistent movement practice.

- Begin to practice the Seven Basic Movement Patterns, focusing on good form as opposed to a high number of repetitions or speed. Know that eventually, you may advance to combinations and compound movements, adding weight, adding repetitions, and ultimately creating comprehensive, total-body workouts that vary throughout the week.

- Acquire or purchase a few pieces of equipment, educational materials, or activewear that can help you on your journey. Start small and be intentional— know that these items are *accessories* to an active lifestyle, not *necessities*.

- While selecting equipment, focus first on minimal, affordable pieces that can serve a multitude of purposes, like a kettlebell, a yoga mat, or a set of dumbbells.

- Begin to utilize your daily movement time and start documenting your feelings postmovement in a journal, on a notepad, or by memory. When you need a boost or encouragement, look back on these reminders for helpful, self-motivated encouragement.

- Engage the senses:
  - Sound—Eliminate noise and turn off podcasts, music, and TV. Listen to the sounds of the environment around you and become comfortable moving in silence.
  - Sight—Instead of looking in the mirror while moving, turn your attention inward and focus on how each movement feels rather than how it looks. If the sights in your workout environment feel like visual noise—as may

be the case in a corporate gym under fluorescent lights—consider taking your workout outdoors or to an uncluttered room filled with natural light. Observe how your visual environment impacts your exercising experience.

- Touch—Pay attention to the nooks and crannies of your body where you hold tension. Focus on these areas as you lift, stretch, or breathe.

Optimize

- You are moving your body every day and have seamlessly integrated movement into your home, work, family, and social life.
- You have come to love, enjoy, and look forward to each opportunity to exercise.
- You have experienced identifiable, measurable positive physical health outcomes.
- You are able to report mental health benefits, such as feeling less anxious or less depressed.
- You have inspired and encouraged others to move with you and are now a point person who can offer guidance for those who are trying to begin implementing a movement culture.
- You have adapted an intergenerational healing mentality. In practice you have included children, pets, and elders in your movement. You view your movement as a chance to break cycles of trauma, to move through hardship, and to build strength that you can pass on to the next generation.

INTERSECTION WITH OTHER CIRCLES

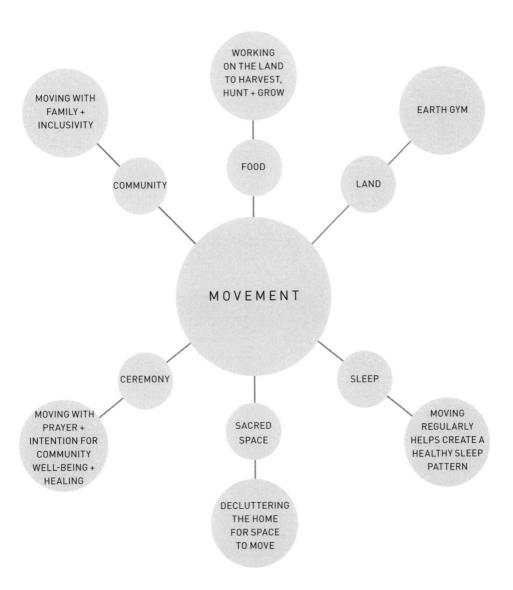

WORKING ON THE LAND TO HARVEST, HUNT + GROW

MOVING WITH FAMILY + INCLUSIVITY

EARTH GYM

FOOD

COMMUNITY

LAND

MOVEMENT

CEREMONY

SLEEP

MOVING WITH PRAYER + INTENTION FOR COMMUNITY WELL-BEING + HEALING

SACRED SPACE

MOVING REGULARLY HELPS CREATE A HEALTHY SLEEP PATTERN

DECLUTTERING THE HOME FOR SPACE TO MOVE

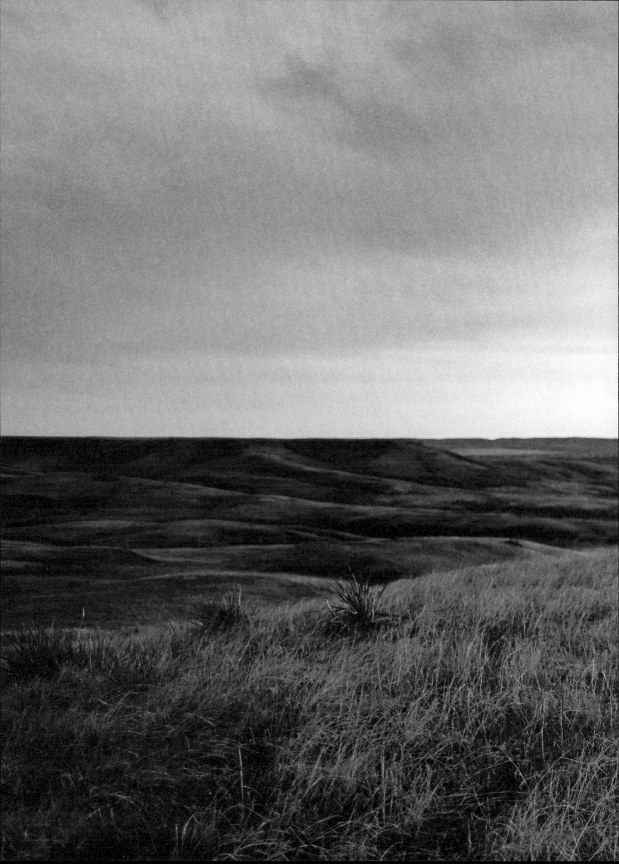

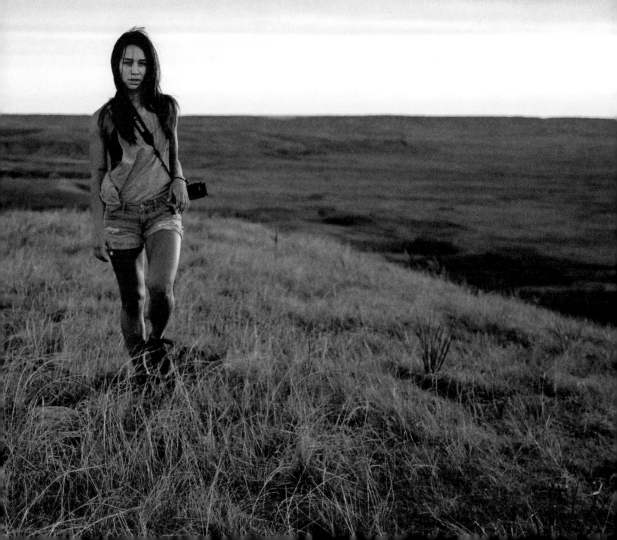

2

LAND

Watch how you walk, you are walking on your mother.

—*Dr. A. C. "Chuck" Ross*

The Lakota believed that all things that helped sustain the body—wind, rain, food, pure air, water, and sun—were medicine.

—*Luther Standing Bear,* Land of the Spotted Eagle

Nothing belongs to us. We are here for the universe. All of us are here to serve the universe.

—*Rita Pitka Blumenstein, in* Grandmothers Counsel the World: Women Elders Offer Their Vision for Our Planet

CULTURE SHIFT:
TOWARD A SUBSISTENCE WORLDVIEW

Indigenous people everywhere share a love and respect for the land. We have never lost this sacred connection. We have never forgotten how Mother Earth provides. Because we understand how much we rely on her, we respect her accordingly. Many view the land as a resource to be used, exploited, owned, and occupied. Indigenous people know that the land is a living entity to have a relationship of respect and reciprocity with. She is life-giver, guardian, the root of all creation, the heart of the universe, and the essence of our very being. When she suffers, so do we. The health of the land is a direct reflection of the health of the people.

Previous spread: Chelsey walks through the West Place, a special part of her family's ranch where she always feels happy to return. Here, she is connected to her Lakota ancestors.

Some Indigenous nations, like the Inuit, still maintain strong subsistence economies, living heavily off of the land despite ongoing environmental degradation. Other nations have been violently removed from their land, animal populations, clean water sources, and subsistence ways of life. But in these instances, they have maintained a *subsistence worldview* as regards the land, which is what we hope for all readers to adopt. This is a critical first step toward improved global health. A subsistence worldview means that we understand how much we rely on the land, and so we respect it and care for it accordingly. Our collective health, and our children's futures, depend on this.

The land is the curator of our original culture, and our reverence for her reflects that. In our creation stories, we emerged from caves, we fell from the sky, and we came to be as a result of interactions and exchanges with the elements, forces of nature, and plant and animal life. Everything we know came to exist this way as well: our languages, our songs, our food systems, our ways of life, our art forms, our intellects, our healing practices, and our spiritual connection. Everything comes from the land. And so, we are taught, the land continues to teach us everything we need to know throughout our lives.

If these ideas sound foreign to you, remember that at one time, in everyone's history, our ancestors were intimately connected to the land. The beautiful and unique aspects of every culture on earth resulted from our interacting with the beautiful, diverse natural regions from where we came. For many, that connection has been severed, and this continues to impact collective health and wellness today. It is imperative that we repair these bonds.

Today, as the climate crisis continues to grow, so do global health crises, as evidenced by the modern prevalence of illnesses like diabetes, heart disease, and cancer. These hardships are interwoven with social ills like displacement, poverty, and inadequate housing. It is no coincidence that as life on earth grows sicker, the root diseases of greed and exploitation continue to damage the very soil, water, and air we humans rely upon.

We have all heard of "Blue Zones"—health hot spots where people are living longer, happier, more fulfilling lives.[1] One of the common themes in Blue Zones

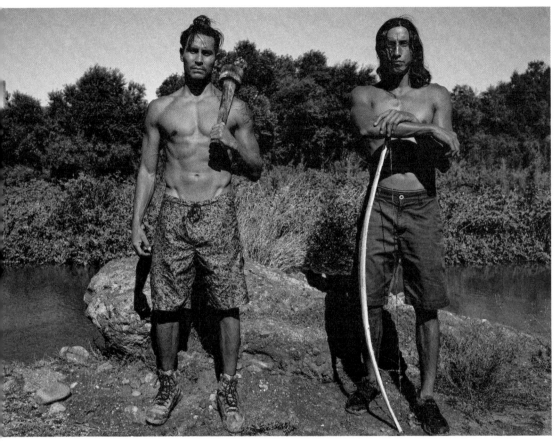

Standing near the On Akimel (Salt River) where they were raised, Thosh (left) and his brother Amson Collins (right) (O'odham, Seneca-Cayuga, Osage) hold a war club and bow, respectively, weapons or tools that their people have always used and that they continue to use today.

is neither technology nor money, but rather that the people in these diverse cultural areas live in harmony with their surroundings and that they are culturally connected. Typically, the United States is not thought of as a hot spot for health. In fact, it is often criticized for its reputation for having a sedentary and overweight population. Of note, the creator of the Blue Zone theory is a Minnesotan. Only two hundred years ago, on the lands we now call Minnesota, it was common for Anishinaabe and Dakota people to live active lives with full mental faculties well past the age of one hundred years. At that time, North America perhaps represented one of the greatest Blue Zones the world has ever seen. It wasn't until the invasion of a land-exploiting culture that this changed. Now, we all have the opportunity to reclaim the Indigenous narrative of good health rather than to accept an unhealthy fate for the people of this land.

This circle of wellness—land, and connection to it—might be viewed as the circle that impacts collective, global health, as opposed to just individual health, more than any other. Indigenous people make up only 5 percent of the world's population, yet they protect 80 percent of the world's biodiversity. This is proof that Indigenous leaders, climate activists, and governments are truly the carriers of the knowledge we need to move forward into a livable, breathable future. We will not pretend to have any answers for solving the climate crisis via technology or policy, but we do have an idea as to how we might begin to effect change from within our hearts and minds, ultimately encouraging more people to care about these issues. It begins with a shift in worldview toward love for the land. Indigenous knowledge may serve as the guide.

Establishing a connection to the land will not only heal our planet, but it will heal our traumas, our spiritual wounds, and our hearts as individuals and families who are seeking to be well. Our ancestors never had to consciously set time aside to connect to the land, because it was simply a part of life. Today, everything we do, from work to recreation, keeps us indoors, often in front of electronic devices that emit unhealthy blue light. Because of this imposed sedentary, indoor culture, we face more illness and more depression, and we feel disconnected from the natural world. We need to consciously reconnect. And once we do, we feel immediate healing benefits that the land provides.

Studies show that as few as five minutes spent outdoors—no matter whether in a city park or deep in a forest—leaves people feeling more positive and boosts self-esteem. Ten minutes spent outdoors on a sunny day boosts our levels of vitamin D—which is critical for keeping our immune systems strong and which many people are deficient in. And twenty minutes outdoors measurably lowers the stress hormone cortisol.[2] If just a few minutes can do all of this, imagine what hours, weeks, and days outdoors would feel like. Imagine a life on the land.

HONOR THE EARTH: CONNECTING TO THE EARTH AND THE ELEMENTS
THOSH

My parents named me Thosh (also spelled T-a-ṣ), which means "sun" in my O'odham language. I come from a place where we are taught to have reverence for the sun. As people of the desert, the sun permeates our landscape.

Many Indigenous people from the southwest engage in morning rituals for acknowledging the sun, which helps us to be grateful for each day of life on Mother Earth. I was taught to stand on the land and face the sun just before it peeks up over the horizon. This time is a sacred time. It is the time of transition between night and day, when the spirits are moving around on the land. As the warm glow of the sun starts to illuminate the eastern mountain ranges, I bring my hands up, palms open, to receive the blessings emitted by the warm glow of dawn. When we bring that glow inward to our chests, we allow the blessing to sink into our hearts. We stand on the land in a mindful way without worrying about what's happening elsewhere, remaining present and grateful for the moment.

As the sun rises above the mountains, rays of light soar across the landscape, transforming it from a place where spirits do their work to one where we two-legged walk. For many, it is this powerful moment that allows the beginning of a sunrise ceremony. *Taṣ tonalig*, the rays of the sun, are powerful gifts. Without these, and other life-giving elements, all life would cease to exist.

All Indigenous people see the earth we walk upon as our mother. All have recognized she is alive and has a spirit. All beings that live on her are manifestations of the work of the Great Creator. And so we thank her. As we stand upon Mother Earth, we stand in a ceremonial way, to acknowledge that she is the one who provides a home for all living beings to walk upon.

Through our words, songs, and actions, we also give thanks to the water for all that it does. Without it, life would cease to exist. We give thanks for the way it cleanses and quenches thirst. We respect water for its life-giving power, as too little or too much of it can kill us. This is why much care is taken when interacting with our relative water.

Air is another powerful gift from Creator that we require every second of our existence. It is constantly around us. It would be easy to take it for granted, but remember it. We can survive days without water and even weeks without food, but we survive only a few moments without oxygen.

Grandfather fire is a relative of the sun. We put our hearts and minds together to give thanks for the warmth of the fire. When we learned to create fire, we became human. We thank the fire for cooking our food, which nourishes our minds, bodies, and spirits. Fire has always had a special role in our ceremonies as the one who burns our medicines, which carry our thoughts and visions of a healthy future into a higher consciousness. The fire creates smoke, which carries the power to bring healing energy to our spaces. Like our relative water, fire is a very powerful creation of the Great Spirit that can heal or destroy in a flash. We respect its power.

Our health is inextricably connected to the natural world in a practical, spiritual way. We live in a very complex, interconnected world of trillions of living organisms, all connected by a source of energy. The spiritual and physical mechanisms that make up all existence are too complex for our human minds to thoroughly grasp, and this is why many of our ancestors described Creator as a great spiritual entity.

If you pay attention, you'll see that all living things in the plant and animal nations have their special roles and their unique ways of ensuring the continuity of life, and they all have their ways of giving thanks. They show us how to play our role in contributing to the balance and harmony of our ecosystem. We need to watch and listen, because right now, humans are different. We are taking too much. The ultimate mark of health and wellness will be a return to balance, reciprocity, and respect for plant life, animal life, the elements, and the earth.

HOW LAND HEALS
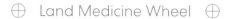
⊕ Land Medicine Wheel ⊕

SPIRITUAL

Spiritual growth and strength cannot be cultivated in a vacuum without a direct connection to the land and elements.

EMOTIONAL

Studies today show what our ancestors have always understood: time spent on the land leads to peacefulness, stress relief, and happiness.

MENTAL

The land is the original curator of our culture, our knowledge, and our traditions. We must once again view the land as our guide, our teacher, and our friend.

PHYSICAL

Human beings evolved to move on the land, no matter the terrain or the weather. Most people today have lost this connection to the outdoors. We must reclaim our relationship to the earth by taking our movement outdoors, once again utilizing our Mother Earth Gym.

THE EARTH IS EVERYWHERE

What do you picture when you hear the word "nature"? Are people around you? Are you near anyone's home? Or have you *escaped* to an area where it's just you and a stunning landscape for your backdrop? The joy and importance of finding silence is undeniable, but there is a danger in the notion that nature exists solely as a pristine, human-free, far-off swath of forest in the middle of a faraway mountain range or national park. When we view nature as a separate or "other" place, off in the distance being preserved by a government entity within a neatly

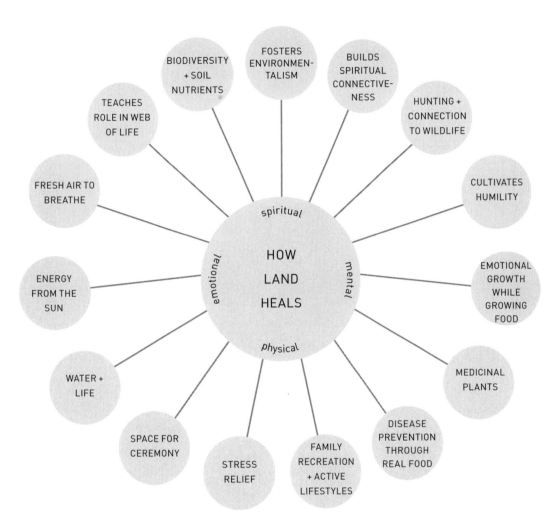

delineated boundary, we support the idea that anything outside of that boundary is somehow *not* nature and therefore is less valuable or worthy of care and preservation. This sets the stage for constant, aggressive, and perhaps even thoughtless urban development.

The capitalist notion of land separates it into two categories—natural and developed. This idea—along with the myth that Indigenous peoples in precontact times lived here and there on a mostly "empty" land that they did "nothing" with—has been one of the most harmful ideas used against Indigenous peoples

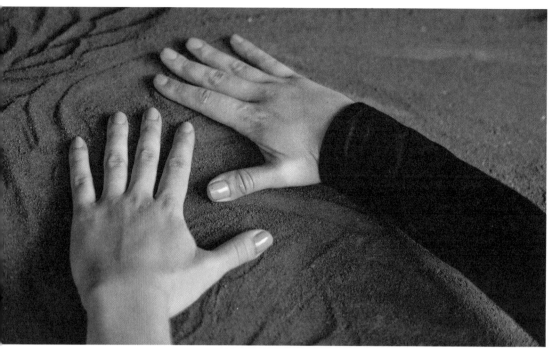

While hiking in a canyon at the foot of Red Mountain, Chelsey enjoys the therapeutic feeling of cool sand on her hands.

throughout history. The myth continues to be part of the American story, used against us as a justification for genocide and the mass land grab, and now used further to mine and exploit our natural resources. Because of this, we personally choose to avoid using the word "nature" at all. Instead, we recognize that the land is everywhere, and we are always on it.

Our ancestors tried to teach early settlers how to live with the land without exploiting it. The settlers certainly took what they needed from this knowledge to survive, but the notion of maintaining restraint did not catch on. We cannot go back and force it, so now that we are here, we have to remember that no matter how many buildings we see, or how much concrete or asphalt surrounds us, we are on and of Mother Earth, and we rely on everything that she provides; thus we are always responsible for taking care of and respecting the land even in places where it seems to be impossible to do so because of development or environmental degradation.

The health of the land is a direct reflection of the health of the people. We cannot get too comfortable with the idea of city, state, and national parks being the only swaths of green space. We need to focus on cleaning up our urban areas, developing more mindfully with eco-friendly architecture and design as a priority, supporting wind and solar technology, preventing pipelines from further contaminating water sources, and taking any other measures to protect the land, air, and water wherever we may be. Environmental health is human health, and so that is why a connection to land plays such a significant role in living a balanced lifestyle.

ON THE LAND, IN NYC
CHELSEY

For a while, I lived in traditional Lenape territory, also known as New York City, and I began to feel disconnected from the earth, from my culture, and from the sense of peace that was once so accessible to me, yet that I had taken for granted while being raised on my Lakota and Anishinaabe homelands in North Dakota. I was finishing grad school and starting my career. I did not have money to spare, so I had no way of traveling outside of the city for fresher air on weekends. One day it finally dawned on me: I didn't have to leave the city to be on the land. I just needed to acknowledge the land all around me and consciously spend time with it, right where I was. So instead of riding the subway, I started to walk.

I'd walk from my apartment in central Brooklyn to the East River waterfront a few miles away. Or after a day of work in a downtown Manhattan office building, I'd window shop through SoHo and then make my way to a museum on the Upper East Side. One weekend, I decided to run. I started at South Street Seaport and ran all the way up the West Side Highway until my feet gave out around 115th Street. I continued this habit of walking and running wherever I could, whenever time permitted, so that I could develop a conception of how much earth I was skipping over when I did in fact ride the train.

This practice completely changed my perspective on New York and made me feel like I understood where I lived like never before. As I walked, I could admire the diversity in appearance and style and attitude of the people whose paths I crossed. I'd visualize the faces, clothing, and foods of the Lenape people who walked here for hundreds of years before it became a city of settlers. I'd go to Prospect Park or Central Park and walk with bare feet—even just a few steps, to feel more grounded. I'd look up at the skyscrapers and visualize the Haudenosaunee ironworkers who have left their legacy there.

It didn't matter that concrete and asphalt surrounded me. I could walk outside. I could breathe fresh air. I could connect to the earth, and I could show respect to the original people who lived in this place. This felt incredibly empowering. And when I'd look up at the sky on a bright sunny day, I'd realized that this was the very same sky and sun that my family was looking at thousands of miles away. We were still connected. Suddenly, I wasn't quite as homesick.

ON THE LAND, IN THE BAY AND LA
THOSH

In 2001, I received the T. C. Cannon Scholarship—a full ride to attend the San Francisco Art Institute, where I went to pursue photography. Many times I found myself running through Golden Gate Park to be among the old-growth trees and away from the hustle and bustle of the city. In the warmer seasons, I hung out at the beach to feel the sun and listen to the water. It reminded me of home.

My roommate Jeremy was Diné, also a nation from the Southwest with a history and strong ongoing heritage of running. At times, we'd run from our apartment in the "Tendernob" to Ocean Beach. We did it partially for cardiovascular fitness and recreation, but more because it was a way for us to maintain our identities and connect to the land we were living on, since we shared a tradition of running being a big part of our identities. We would also go across the Golden

Gate Bridge to regularly hike in the Muir Woods. While driving back to the city, I would look over Ohlone territory—now known as San Francisco—and I would try to imagine how it might have been before Spanish and American settlers began occupying and changing the ecology of the land.

In 2005, when I moved to Tongva territory—now known as Los Angeles—I had the same reverence for the undeveloped places of the region. In those days it was not really on my radar to learn about the wild foods of the region. My connection to the land as a visitor was predominantly rooted in having respect for it and appreciating the peaceful energy it contributed to my well-being. Wherever I traveled in Turtle Island—a commonly used Indigenous name for North America—expressing a reverence for the land and minimizing my footprint was a value I carried, which ultimately led me back to my home.

I moved back to Salt River in 2011, which was the plan all along. Growing up connected to the land, I always knew where my home was and that I was merely going off for a while to explore the world. In retrospect, I think I was subconsciously trying to fulfill a temporarily missing component that existed in the original Indigenous protocols, where young men went on a faraway journey to gain knowledge after their coming-of-age ceremony.

Just before I went away to college, I was at a gathering on the rez, and one of our elder spiritual leaders approached me and said, "When you go there, never forget who you are. I'll pray for you." She said this in very simple terms, but with her tone and the stern look in her eyes, it seemed like she transmitted an energy to my consciousness that communicated to me how imperative it was that I stay on a good path and watch out for all the challenges that I would face in the city.

Everywhere I have traveled in Native Country I've heard elders say that if you go away, never forget who you are and where you come from. Always learn what you can, but then come back home and help contribute to the community with the knowledge you have learned during your time away.

᭡

We learned a lot from our parallel experiences as rez kids who grew up with strong connections to the land but then moved away to big cities. First, we realized what a gift it was to be raised with creation stories, ceremonies, and culture that kept us connected to, rooted in, and respectful of our stunningly beautiful homelands—the Great Plains and the Sonoran Desert. Then, by experiencing life far away from these places, we realized the degree to which we missed these deeply engrained parts of ourselves and how simply being in a faraway environment can impact your mood and sense of self. Most important, we learned that land heals, no matter where you are. As each of us, in our own time and in our own world, figured out how to apply our ancestral teachings to life in the big city, we experienced growth, nurturing, and a sense of much-needed peace.

YOU HAVE A PLACE YOU CAN RETURN TO: CEREMONIAL CONNECTIONS TO LAND

Although our daughters are too young to understand it, we have already begun to guide them in establishing a connection to the land by rooting them home ceremonially. Both of their placentas are buried on our land, right next to each other, near our field where we grow squash, corn, and beans. When we buried their placentas, we gathered with our family, offered tobacco and songs, and said words of thanks for their lives and spirits. We prayed that as they continue to grow, they will always know that they have a home. We also prayed that they will adapt these teachings of love and respect for the land and learn to take care of Mother Earth.

As we pray for these things, we know that this ask comes with personal responsibility. It is up to us to continue to educate our daughters every day in our ancestral ways and to work to give them these values in a world that does not always demonstrate the same. From time to time, we point out to them the place where their placentas are buried, and we tell them all about the ceremony and its meaning. The ceremony will live on as a story, becoming a formative pillar to help them understand who they are.

Placenta burial is a ceremony that is seen across many, but not all, tribes, and each nation and family has its own way of doing it. The symbolism in the ceremony is profound, as are the stories that will follow it. These stories will become a piece of our children's lives that will help them realize who they are and understand their place in the world. We must consciously guide our children toward a connection to the land from the time that they are born, because we know that the land will continue to take care of them. In this way, we are instilling in our children a feeling of reciprocity and responsibility for giving back to the earth for what it provides. We are showing them that they are literally a part of the land.

LOVE THE LAND, LOVE YOUR DESCENDANTS
CHELSEY

I never heard the word "wellness" growing up. But I unwittingly developed a deep understanding of wellness by way of being raised with my traditional Lakota spirituality and would later connect the dots when the wellness conversation became mainstream, which happened around the same time I quit drinking and started taking my health into my own hands in a meaningful way.

When I was a kid, my parents never explicitly instructed me to care about the earth. I don't recall having conversations with my family about environmentalism or recycling or the size of my carbon footprint. Most families were not having such conversations in the early 1990s. Yet just as my spiritual teachings anchored the roots of my wellness worldview, the seeds of my environmentalism had been planted by Indigenous teachings long before talk of saving the planet began to hit the mainstream. I already understood the importance of the earth and elements in a meaningful way, because the significance of the land was deeply engrained in my worldview by way of prayer.

Growing up, I learned to pray from the perspective of the Lakota worldview. As a child who was exposed to both Catholicism and Lakota spirituality, I recall thinking that the Lakota way was easy to understand, was practical, and made so much sense. The essence of this worldview is rooted in the land. The way that we prayed, the words that we said when we prayed, the things we prayed for, the places where we prayed, and the medicines that we burned to pray with—all of these involved the natural world around us.

When I pray today, I think about the plant nations that help us by providing nourishing foods and healing medicines. They give us the building blocks to create fire, and they carry our prayers and cleanse our space with their smoke. I think of the winged nations, the eagles and hawks who have dropped their feathers to help us find our way and to remind us who we are—two-legged people who walk the earth. I think of the thunder being nation, which brings renewal in the springtime and provides water for us throughout life, and how without water we would not be here. The thunder beings remind us that seasons of life will always change, and if times are hard now, they will be good again later. I think of the buffalo nation, which provides shelter and food. I think of all of the life-giving elements and beings from all four directions—red, yellow, black, white—who all serve a purpose and play a role in all aspects of mental, physical, spiritual, and emotional life. I think of the interconnectedness of all things, and I wonder how I can play a role in this web of life. How can I be more helpful than harmful? I think about balance, and I ask for guidance in maintaining it.

Because I learned to pray this way, and to acknowledge everything that brings life, I learned to view the world through a lens of gratitude for all living things, for all parts of the land, for all people, and for all of creation. I learned not to discriminate, not to view myself or any part of humanity as being above or superior to other life on earth. This is why I have reverence for the land.

As a person who is deeply concerned for the well-being of future generations, I consider it my responsibility to teach my children to pray this way and to raise them with this worldview. In Lakota spirituality we call it *mitakuye oyasin*—we are all related. We are to work with and alongside our relatives—human, plant, animal, and elemental—so that we can set up a good future for our descendants. I will never meet them and I will never know them, but they occupy a special place in my heart. Everyone should love their descendants, and caring for the land is one way of expressing this love.

FAMILY AND COMMUNITY CONNECTION TO LAND
THOSH

My first real connection to the land started with the river that runs through our reservation. The Ce:dagĭ Akimel (Verde River) and On Akimel (Salt River) converge within our borders and continue through the community and into the city. For thousands of years these two rivers have been the lifelines of the people, animals, and plants who have inhabited the region now known as the Phoenix metropolitan area. The Hekiokam (people who lived long ago), also known as the Hohokam, lived all across the Sonoran Desert, as far south as northern Mexico, as well as in this region along the Ce:dagĭ and On Akimel. They were masters of their environment, achieving economic stability and environmental sustainability in this hot, dry climate for millennia. They are known for building extensive and elaborate canal systems. The Hekiokam, who built the canals and other technology required to irrigate desert crops, are the ancestors of the O'odham people who live today.

Our spiritual leaders say that the area where the two rivers converge is a place that holds power. While I was growing up on the rez, cultural leaders speaking at community gatherings would always remind us about the importance of the river and how it is a powerful resource that we must continue to cherish and take care of. I imagine that our political leaders in the late 1800s, while negotiating treaties and rights to land, must have understood this and made it a point to fight for the river convergence to be included within our reservation borders. The United States government unfairly seized millions of acres of O'odham land, but

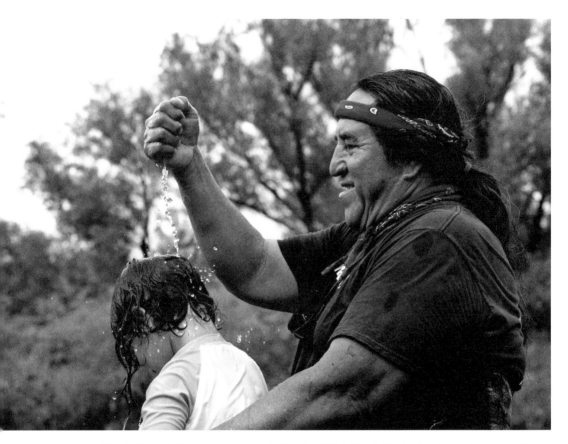

Tony Collins and Alo enjoy playtime in the On Akimel (Salt River). The land and water bring joy and healing to their family.

the river convergence and a few other locations of spiritual reverence remained ours.

When I became initiated into the spiritual runners group in 1991, I started to understand the river as a place of reverence, not just of recreation. Out of respect for community privacy, I won't share too many details, though it is important to mention because it is a formative memory that set me on a good path for the rest of my life.

We camped there for four days and nights, and we fasted. At sunrise on the fourth morning, we were instructed to get in the water. It was a cold November morning, about forty degrees. I was shivering uncontrollably and feeling tired and hungry, dreaming of the comfort of my bedroom and a hot meal cooked by my mom. But there I was. I took my time creeping into the water while the men, like my dad, went crashing right in. Finally I jumped in and struggled to catch my breath because of the cold. Our cultural leaders explained to us that we were cleaning ourselves and getting power from the river in preparation for the long run ahead of us. This experience was hard, but it gave me a real sense of belonging, and to my surprise, it really did help me run! I felt strong and proud, and I was glad I had done it. Looking back, I now know that jumping into that freezing water meant more than just being tough—it was about consciously increasing grit and durability, and developing a connection to the river, to one another, and to the elements.

From then on, my view of the river and the importance of sacred sites and my homelands was forever expanded. But I'd be lying if I said I never took it for granted. There was a time, in my late teens and early twenties, when I got caught up in city life, and all I wanted to do was go to raves, clubs, and parties. When my dad would ask me to help him harvest wood or hunt in the desert, I'd be itching to leave after a few hours, worried I was missing out on something with my friends. But after a few years of living that lifestyle—which could be very unforgiving—I started to remember how much I loved and missed my homelands, and I started to realize how much I had taken my connections to land and culture for granted.

The fact that the land eventually called me back is proof of the power of our ancestral teachings, our ceremonies, and our land. When I was ready to return, I felt comforted, loved, and grateful knowing that the land and my family had been there waiting for me all along. One time, when I was living in California working as a photographer, I returned home for a weekend during late summer. As I drove in, the sun was rising and I could smell the fresh scent of rain mixed with ṣeg:oi (greasewood). I knew then that I would move back. And when I did, I not only committed to reconnecting with my land and community, but also to reciprocating all that they had given me. If I do my part in taking care of the land, it will continue to take care of me in return.

Today, living again on my ancestral land, I have my own family, and it is my role to facilitate our connection to the land. My parents raised my siblings and me by taking us to the river and out on the land, and now Chelsey and I have the chance to continue fostering that relationship for Alo and Westyn. We keep connected through the O'odham foodways of foraging, hunting, and farming. From time to time we try to take our workouts outside among the elements—into the Earth Gym. We make it a point to get away from the city and visit the river or the nearby desert preserve to enjoy the peace it has to offer. Many times this is something as simple as walking through the desert exploring with our girls, observing the desert animals, and letting them develop footing and spatial awareness that is necessary for safely hiking around the rugged terrain. It is a critical piece to our total well-being.

Making these regular visits to the desert is the norm for Alo. As we write this, she is only a toddler, but she has been to areas of the desert that many people in her own community have never seen. (Because of traumas and other hardships that our people experience, many of them, even from the same rez as us, have not had the cultural privilege of establishing a connection to the land like we have.) This makes me feel all the more grateful to have the opportunity to raise her this way. We do not take it for granted. One day, around the time when Alo was just learning to talk, she and I went to visit the river. As we walked up to its banks, she looked up at me and said, "Wooow, is pwetty Dada." That made my heart so happy, because she recognized what is real and what matters in our world. It also affirmed my understanding that even as babies, our children absorb so much, and they are never too young to get to know the land.

Whenever an O'odham social dance or some kind of ceremony is happening, we try our best to attend in order to strengthen our spiritual health and connect with extended family in the community. Since gatherings always happen outside, this is also another way to strengthen connection to the land.

We do all of these activities in order to maintain and grow our relationship to the land as a family. We are building upon the things we were taught growing up. Inevitably, when we are out there, Chelsey also brings up stories about the land where she comes from, what it was like for her to get to know those areas as a child, what she knows of her family's and nation's history on her land, and how it relates to our teachings in the desert. It is all connected. We are revitalizing certain Indigenous lifeways that were nearly lost because of colonialism. All the while, we give ourselves permission to evolve cultural practices that meet our needs here and now.

With every generation we must become more connected to the land and have more accessibility to Indigenous food practices and knowledge than the generation before. It starts with us, here and now. Many people in my generation in Indian Country from reservations everywhere are working to revitalize, preserve, and evolve our Indigenous lifeways. It is with this understanding that our connection to land, food, movement, ceremony, family, and community all intersect with concepts such as intergenerational thinking and cultural regeneration to make up the foundation of our Indigenous lifeways that give us purpose in the world.

Now, whenever I have the chance, I share with the people of my community my views on the importance of maintaining and strengthening a connection to the bit of land we have left. The well-being of the people, the animals, the plants, and the entire land base depends on how much we value that land. It provides cultural and spiritual privacy. It offers food by way of foraging, hunting, and fishing. It offers a place of family gathering for sociability and ceremony. I believe that our ancestral reverence for the land should be reflected within the policies and governments of all Native communities and beyond.

We are fortunate to have a river that runs through our reservation. Considering how hard it can be to live in the desert, even with modern conveniences, you can understand why preindustrial peoples regarded the river as sacred. We cannot forget that it is still the lifeline of the people. There are many great teachings to gain from pondering this concept.

Every aspect of the Seven Circles of Wellness can be viewed as templates to establish a connection to the land. You can eat from the land, sleep outside, take your workouts outside, and spend time with family and community through ceremonial or social gatherings. Being present while on the land helps you to realign with Mother Earth's frequency and to heal from the hustle and bustle of the modern world.

TAKE ACTION: HOW TO CONNECT TO THE LAND

Learn

· Shift your worldview: the land is not a separate entity "out there" in "nature." You are always on the land.

· The land takes care of you, not the other way around. Learn to respect the land accordingly.

· Identify and acknowledge the Indigenous territory on which you live.

· Get to know your sacred landmarks and areas of spiritual significance, and the oral tradition, histories, and stories that go with them.

· Learn about the plants, animals, and wildlife that surround you.

· Identify foods that you can hunt, forage, and grow in your area.

Engage

· Begin to observe seasonal changes and inherent characteristics of your environment, including animal behavior, plant behavior, weather patterns, sunrise and sunset, moon cycles, solstice, and equinox.

· Use all five senses to connect to the natural elements of your environment—what do you see, hear, taste, smell, and feel?

· Take your training outdoors and engage in Earth Gym.

· With respectful protocols at the forefront, begin engaging with outdoor food processes such as harvesting, gathering, fishing, and hunting.

· Sleep outdoors at least a few times a year—observe the changes in your circadian rhythm, how different it feels when you sleep under the stars and wake up with the sunrise.

· Acknowledge all of the life-giving elements from all directions and honor them.

Optimize

· You have learned to fully respect, appreciate, and honor the land that you walk upon, and you consider it your relative, not just an object or a resource to be used for commercial or development purposes.

· You have integrated food practices like gathering wild foods or growing herbs in your windowsill—these are the things you look forward to, a part of your daily culture.

· The holidays you celebrate are not just commercial—they now include harvesting, planting, equinox, solstice, and other markers that demonstrate a connection to the natural world.

- You can reflect upon and report positive impacts on your well-being; you can interpret your personal experiences, feelings, and observances to others; and you can share stories about the ways that your connection to land has grown and helped you.
- You can now reflect positively on your sense of belonging and your understanding of your role in the land and the larger ecosystem of living organisms.

Intersection with Other Circles

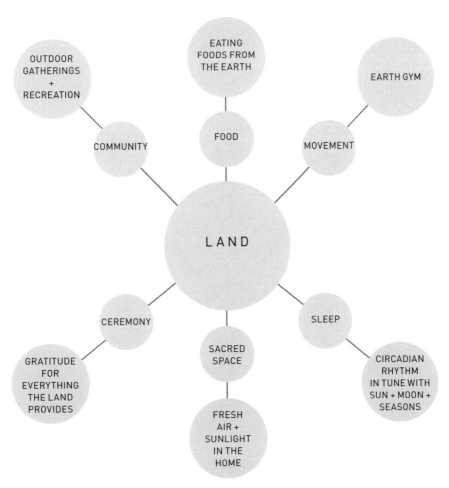

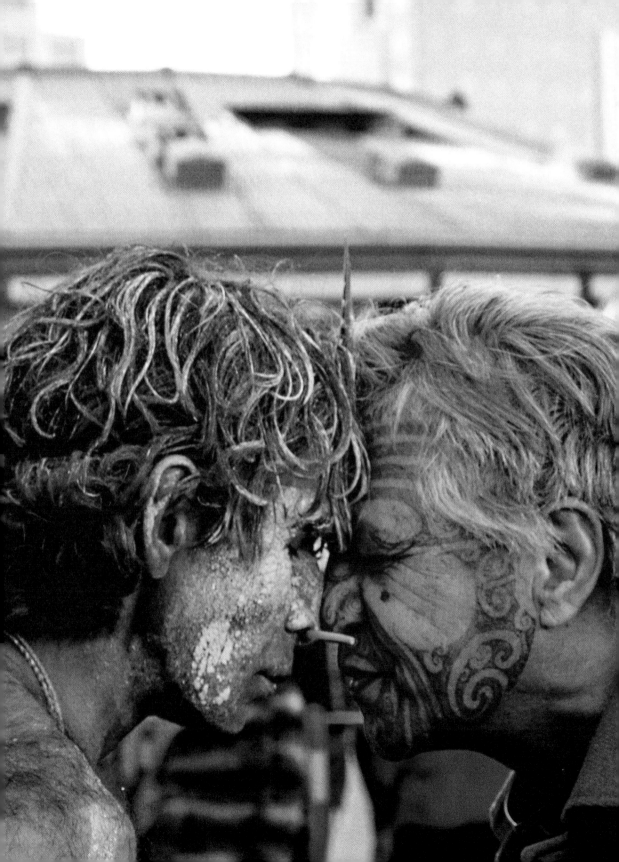

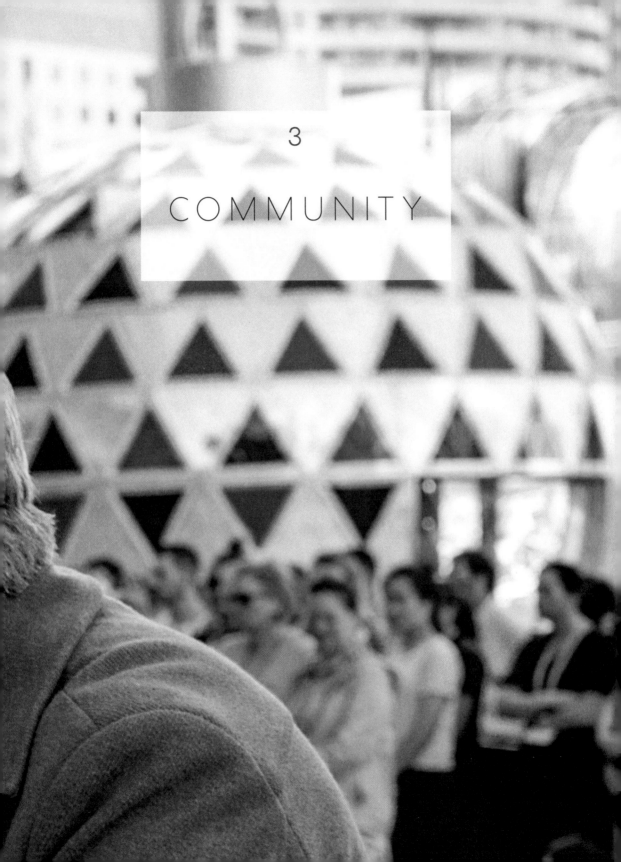

3

COMMUNITY

The ultimate aim of life, stripped of accessories, was quite simple:
One must obey kinship rules; one must be a good relative.

—Ella Deloria (Dakota anthropologist), Waterlily

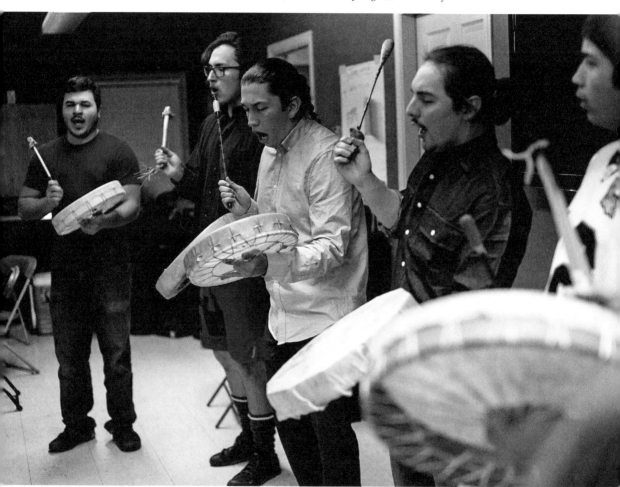

Khelsilem (Squamish), third from left, a community leader and language instructor, sings a song with their peers in the Skwxwu7mesh language.

Previous spread: Les McLeod, an Aboriginal dancer in traditional paint and regalia (left), and a Maori elder (right) exchange a traditional Maori greeting of respect called "sharing breath" at the Healing Our Spirits Worldwide conference.

KINSHIP AND CONNECTION

At a powwow in Southern California, where hundreds of dancers from dozens of nations came to compete, we watched as a young boy, maybe twelve years old, won his first grass dancing contest. Over the microphone, the announcer proclaimed his victory. He smiled big as he received his cash prize of several hundred dollars from the judges. A new set of dancers entered the arena, and the next event started. But we kept our eyes on the boy and watched him walk to the sidelines, where the drum groups sat. He found the crew who had sung as he danced. He placed his entire envelope of earnings on the center of their big drum and shook hands with each singer. He left his reward but came away with something greater. He showed the world that his family had taught him to be generous.

At any kind of Indigenous community event, one will notice these moments of kinship magic that take place throughout. Humble demonstrations of respect, honor, dignity, and unconditional love from relative to relative abound. Our extended family ties remain remarkably strong and have carried us and our cultural practices through the innumerable hardships we have experienced over the past few generations. Our community values are unforgotten and steadfast, hardly tarnished by the perils of colonialism. These values remain the roots that allow all other aspects of our cultural revitalization and health reclamation to grow.

In Native communities, elders are always prioritized and included. Children are welcomed and celebrated. Babies are completely and utterly adored. Cousins look after cousins. Sisters take care of brothers. From the time they are born, Indigenous children are taught and reminded that they are a part of something larger than themselves, that their actions affect those around them, that they have the responsibility to pave a good path for future generations, and that they are honoring their ancestors by honoring kinship values.

The unique and heightened ways that Indigenous people uphold community are so deeply engrained that Native communities can indeed serve as examples to others who seek to bolster their own relationships, families, and connections in life. At the end of the day, while Indigenous communities continue to suffer from loss of land, from discrimination, and from other residual social ills related to colonialism, community and connection keep us functioning, striving, and hoping for a better future. When food options are lacking, when the gym is run down, when the education system is failing, and when the economy is a disaster, this sense of community remains. Like the land, like the elements, like the other foundational pieces of life that we rely on to maintain life itself, community is a central component to well-being, for Indigenous communities and beyond.

Most people today are unaware of the toll that a lack of connection is taking on our health. In the 1980s, only 20 percent of Americans reported being lonely, but today, that number has risen to nearly 50 percent. Studies have pointed to isolation as a root cause of many diseases and health problems, leading to increased risk for disrupted sleep, heightened blood pressure, stroke, declining brain function, depression, and anxiety. What's more, lack of social connection can lead to inflammation, weakened immune systems, and ultimately, shorter lifespans. Some are calling loneliness and disconnection the biggest health problem in America today, more than obesity, smoking, or heart disease.[1] But the good news is that social connections can be nurtured and rebuilt. Now that we know how important community is, we can center it once again. Not only is this possible, it is needed.

Too often, we think of self-care as selfish, and we think of exercise and healthy eating as extracurricular activities. We guilt ourselves into viewing these efforts as an unfair use of our time or budget, or as something that takes us away from our families. What's more, we remain so absorbed in the digital world that we fail to nurture real-life connections with the people around us.

It is time to save community. Everyone can understand and be fulfilled by their role in a greater network. We all have an opportunity to give more to others, to do more good, and to impact our personal and family health by refocusing on community health. For emotional well-being, for a sense of safety and comfort, for a clear sense of identity, and for a clear understanding of our role in life, we rely on community. Fostering healthy relationships, honoring reciprocity, and understanding the ripple effect that our behavior has on the world—all are actions that create collective well-being. Being a part of community is not just for fun; it is vital to our health.

Through the Seven Circles of Wellness, we can learn how to incorporate community holistically. We lift weights so that we can lift babies. We sit on the earth to pray and be mindful so that we can develop a relationship to the land, which heals our spirit while simultaneously leading us toward a commitment to protecting the environment. We grow, hunt, harvest, and prepare food in reciprocity with plant and animal life so that we can provide nourishment for our friends and relatives. We raise our hands in gratitude for the abundance that surrounds us, and we raise our fists in solidarity with progressive social justice movements so that we can raise our children in a better world. Human beings are humble singularities made great by our connection to an unending web of other seen and unseen, living and unliving entities. Anyone can picture an image of support surrounding them and allow a feeling of immense comfort to take hold, balanced by a sense of great responsibility. The health of the self ripples outward and becomes the health of the people. Wellness is never a solo journey, because we are all connected and related.

What is the point of our personal wellness if not for the betterment of others? Healthy people make healthy families, healthy families make healthy communities, and healthy communities make a stronger, safer, cleaner, more balanced world. Contrary to what the wellness industry will tell you, the pursuit of health is not about good looks, image, or social status. Contrary to what patriarchal systems have demonstrated throughout history, the building of strength is not about overpowering others. Instead, the Indigenous perspective on health is one that is focused on healing from within in order to cause a positive outward ripple effect, contributing to a greater good and redistributing strength. Creating community is wellness.

The work of healing is daunting at times. It is a nonlinear path that can feel endless and hard, especially if we think of it as an individual mission. But when we center community, when we realize that we have a responsibility to be well for others, and when we understand that we have the ability to affect future generations in a positive way, suddenly the work begins to make sense and fall into place naturally. We become more motivated than ever to prioritize our health when we realize that our own efforts can make an impact. We are always a part of something greater than ourselves.

Community is a critical piece to living a balanced life because it gives individuals a purpose, and it provides people with a role, which leads to feeling motivated, important, and driven. Anyone who has ever felt a sense of loss or confusion while unemployed or while going through the growing pains of adolescence knows how good it feels to finally find your path. Kinship gives us a sense of responsibility for others, which in turn fosters self-worth, belonging, leadership, empathy, confidence, and compassion. It feels good to fulfill the needs of others who rely on you, whether they are your children, parents, or colleagues. It feels great to be a source of strength whom others come to for guidance and help. There is a delicate balance of independence and interdependence that all people must learn in order to grow with healthy boundaries, healthy relationships, and the ability to contribute fairly while not being taken advantage of. Consciously navigating through the nuances of community and family helps us to develop a sense of this balance. We must raise our children in community once again.

Community extends beyond our present-day, immediate social and familial networks. The Indigenous worldview of community includes our ancestors and our descendants. It is intergenerational. By following this definition of community and kinship, we can remain simultaneously connected to the past, present, and future. We can learn from history, we can contribute to the present, and we can set the stage for a better future. Today, still, a commitment to community is not an entirely selfless pursuit. We must remember that we rely on our communities just as much as they rely on us. On our wellness journeys, we must stay humble and remember that without relationships, we are nothing.

HOW COMMUNITY HEALS
⊕ Community Medicine Wheel ⊕

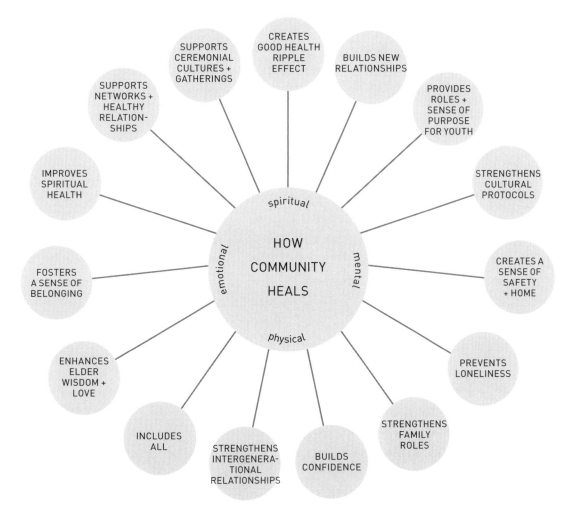

SPIRITUAL

Indigenous spirituality centers community over the self, because we are nothing and no one when we are not in relation to other people, beings, and entities.

EMOTIONAL

Intricate Indigenous kinship and clanship systems have worked brilliantly to ensure that each individual and family knows their role and their place in the community at large, leading to feelings of self-worth and a state of self-actualization. Today, we may once again ensure that our children walk in this world with a sense of knowing who they are and how they can contribute, preventing them from feeling lost or hopeless. This requires a shift toward ancestral parenting and educational methods, in which mentorship, gentle guidance, and doing are utilized instead of harsh discipline, shame, and telling.

MENTAL

Our ancestors always governed and led their families with community at the center of decision-making, leading to societies where thorough community deliberation led to little conflict and lives of peace. Today, we may understand once again that when posed with challenges of the mind, we may ask for help and guidance. Not only is it okay to not know the answers, it is honorable. We may also remember to honor the knowledge and wisdom of babies and elders, those whose spirits are closest to Creator. This form of wisdom is often missing from modern societies—a missed opportunity for mental clarity and growth.

PHYSICAL

As individuals, we are all one small piece of creation, and what we do for our wellness has a ripple effect throughout the world. We all have a duty to be good relatives to one another and to the physical world around us—the land, water, mountains, air, forests, animals, plants, and unseen beings. When we remember that we are in community with the entire world, and we all focus on how our own actions affect the health of everything around us, we create a healthier environment on which our physical health may thrive once again.

COMMUNITY TEACHINGS FROM OUR NATIONS

The importance of community and kinship is not the same in every Indigenous nation, but it is something that nearly every tribal community expresses in its own unique and profound way. All of these values are not just precolonial, but contemporary as well. Here we share some of the core community values from each of our tribal nations that continue to inform our understanding of health and wellness today.

THOSH

ACCOUNTABILITY: I learned that when we walk in the world and come across women who are of the same generation as our mother, we treat them with the same respect. When we come across young men or women who are of the same generation as ourselves, we treat them as our kin. When we come across children who are the same age as our nieces and nephews or our own children, we treat them as our own, whether we know them or not. This is a basic guideline for how to be a good citizen of a nation or community. It prevents violence and conflict. It keeps everyone protected. This value needs to be instilled and fostered at an early age so that it becomes the norm for our children.

I was told that when you are in the community, your actions, good and bad, reflect your family. When you are in Native Country, your actions reflect your tribal nation. When you go outside of Native Country into the dominant society, your actions reflect all Native people. This is a huge responsibility to shoulder, but the trade-off is that it is also a great privilege to be viewed as kin by all Native people. It is not a bad thing to be held accountable. It shows that you belong. Keeping this in mind teaches how to walk in a good way.

S'VAGIMA—TO BE INDUSTRIOUS (O'ODHAM): The O'odham are a farming people who once cultivated massive fields of crops as families, which is how we made a living in precolonial times. It is important to be resourceful and hardworking so that others can rely on you, rather than you relying on others. This brings honor to the home. Within this value, it is said that one should never borrow things from others, but rather should work hard to have one's own tools and supplies. Everyone carried themselves in this way in the early days, and that is how we were able to survive in the desert where life can be hard.

EÑ-I:BDAGĬ AMJED HIM[2]—TO WALK FROM MY HEART (O'ODHAM): To walk from the heart means that we should allow our heart to be the leading force that guides us through life. We treat others how we wish to be treated. We lead with compassion. The cultural leader Serena Padilla expresses this simply: "We put out to the community what we want to get back for ourselves and our families." We hold ourselves accountable, and we have others to hold us accountable as well, which gives us purpose and footing.

DEHORNING (HAUDENOSAUNEE): From my maternal lineage, I am Seneca, which is one of the nations within the Haudenosaunee Confederacy. From this side of my teachings, I have learned that each chief, when appointed, is given horns to wear as a part of his regalia. The horns represent the deer, who uses his horns as a sensory tool. Tom Porter, a well-respected Haudenosaunee elder, has said that when a chief wears horns, he has a heightened sense of awareness and is better able to see, hear, feel, and understand, which is critical for serving the people. If the chief acts dishonorably or fails to live up to his commitment to his community, the clan mothers will dehorn him. When a chief is dehorned, blood drips into his eyes and he can no longer see clearly. He will then sit with his feet dangling from the edge of the earth with no footing.[3] This exemplifies how seriously our people have always taken our responsibilities toward community. When we fail to live up to our commitment to our people, we may harm others or cause disruption, but above all, we harm ourselves.

CHELSEY

MITAKUYE OYASIN—WE ARE ALL RELATED (LAKOTA): The Lakota phrase *mi-takuye oyasin* loosely translates as "we are all related" or "all my relations" (of course, it is far more involved than what the English translation suggests). This phrase represents the essence of our worldview and the basis of our spiritual education. It demonstrates that a broad vision of kinship sits at the core of Lakota values and beliefs. *Mitakuye oyasin* recognizes that everything and everyone, from human to plant to animal life and even the earth and universe, are related. We are all connected. All entities—people, stalks of corn, stars in the sky, rocks on the ocean floor—are equally important and equally insignificant. To understand *mitakuye oyasin* is to take on responsibility for every action and decision in life. When one is raised with this value, it is a given that one must act in such a way that helps rather than harms. It is understood that our actions impact the entire world.

SEVEN GRANDFATHERS TEACHINGS (ANISHINAABE/OJIBWE): The Seven Grandfathers Teachings are a set of values conceptualized in precolonial times, and they remain central to the culture of Anishinaabe and Cree–Metis people. The teachings are widely taught at schools and in homes, and most important they are exemplified through the actions of leaders and parents. The seven teachings are:

1. *Gwayakwaadiziwin* (Honesty): To be sincere and fair in every circumstance.
2. *Debwewin* (Truth): To be loyal and honest to the best of one's abilities.
3. *Inendizowin* (Humility): To be empathetic, compassionate, and respectful of others. To know one's place as a small but equal part of creation. To recognize one's own weaknesses but also one's capacity for growth. To listen and observe.
4. *Zaagi'idiwin* (Love): To demonstrate kindness, compassion, acceptance, and a commitment to working cooperatively with others. To be hopeful and inspiring.
5. *Nibwaakaawin* (Wisdom): To be reflective. To be a seeker of knowledge and

guidance from elders and teachers. To appreciate the opportunity to learn. To be persistent in improving and learning.

6. *Zoongide'iwin* (Courage): To be brave and strong. To acknowledge and accept one's own weaknesses. To take initiative.

7. *Manaaji'idiwin* (Respect): To accept and embrace cultural, religious, and identity differences. To uphold the rights and individuality of others in high esteem. To carry oneself with dignity.[4]

FOSTERING A SACRED CIRCLE OF HEALTHY RELATIONSHIPS

We hear that in the old days, healthy relationships based on equality and mutual respect were the norm. With the influence of Western patriarchy, the culture of healthy relationships has been disrupted. Today, we must remember what a healthy relationship looks like, and we must learn to expect and cultivate these types of relationships for ourselves. Whether we are talking about partnerships, marriages, friendships, the relationship between co-workers or between guardian and child, or any other type of relationship, it is important to recognize some basic principles of what these should look like. Being part of a healthy relationship and a network of support can make all the difference in one's ability to thrive and live in balance in all other areas. Abusive and toxic relationships can be powerful enough to completely degrade one's health. Unfortunately, these types of relationships have become so normal that it can sometimes be difficult to recognize them, even if we are in the midst of one.

Many of us grow up seeing unhealthy relationships, so we can begin this journey by educating ourselves on what a healthy relationship looks like. Traits of a healthy relationship include the following:

- Each person is independent and makes life easier for the other, not harder.
- An idea of commitment is shared and agreed upon.
- Open communication is consistently evaluated and reprioritized.
- Each person's strengths are appreciated and acknowledged.
- Each person clearly understands, acknowledges, and feels good about their role in the relationship.
- Each person feels valued and needed.
- Each person is respected and treated as sacred.
- Trust is paramount for all parties.
- Love and positive feedback are abundant.

Beyond cultivating individual healthy relationships, you can aim to establish a network of support that we call a *sacred circle*. You know that you have a sacred circle when you get to a place in life where you can confidently look around and identify a handful of people with whom you have healthy relationships. This is something to celebrate, to cherish, and to never take for granted. Make it your life's mission to continually feed and grow this sacred circle. This is how deeper happiness and meaning in life are reached—when we are lovingly bonded to those around us; when we are both receiving and contributing good energy, conversation, support, and emotional nurturing.

Sometimes it is necessary to draw boundaries, sever ties, or find other ways to keep your circle protected. It is never easy to discern who should not be in your circle, because often it is a beloved family member who is suffering from trauma and acting in a way that does not serve you or others. We can have compassion for this while also drawing boundaries—a difficult yet important wellness tool that will allow you to maintain distant relationships with some, while keeping your closest loved ones safely within. Your circle will ebb and flow as life goes on. This is normal and okay. With constant attention, at some point, it will feel relatively consistent and steady. When it does, observe how this network of solid support impacts your health in positive ways.

INDIGENOUS LEARNING

Shift the mindset from "My child is disrupting my job and work-flow" to "my job and capitalism are disrupting my connection with my child," because children are not the disruption.

—*Andrea Landry (Anishinaabe), writer and educator*

Indigenous approaches to community as a pillar of well-being permeate every phase of life, and nothing captures this ethos like our precolonial philosophies on teaching and learning. In the old days, every Indigenous nation maintained integrative education systems that were seamlessly woven into kinship structures and families. Rather than shuffling all children into an identical course of learning, each child was recognized for their individuality and was celebrated for their particular gifts. Parents, uncles, aunties, and grandparents contributed to their education. Life was a constant job shadow, where every adult taught and every child learned. Educational duties fell on the collective. Elders taught oral tradition, spiritual wisdom, history, manners, and etiquette. Parents taught household duties and foodways and were responsible for facilitating an emotionally safe environment. Uncles or older boys taught how to hunt, fish, and make tools and weaponry. Aunties taught artistic skills, butchery, hide tanning, construction of homes, and sewing. Each child was given an opportunity to chart their own course for specialization. They were given the freedom to choose their own mentors and guides.

Adults typically did not talk much while teaching, but rather demonstrated and included. Oral tradition says that the collective "sixth sense" was much stronger in the old days, which means that instead of relying solely on speech and words, all people developed a heightened awareness through the use of the other senses. It would have been considered deeply shameful to exclude a child or leave a child feeling lost and without a role. It was in everyone's interest to ensure that all children were lovingly educated.

This structure is quite different from the American educational system, where each child is taught the same set of skills on a rigid timeline in competition with other children. It is a system that takes place in a box, and within that box there are more boxes: square classrooms, square desks, square papers, and square folders that keep each subject compartmentalized and separated from everything else. In this system, certain children (or even entire communities of children) thrive while others are left behind, and when they do fail, it is considered an individual failure. American schools are in a separate environment from the home, away from the family and other relatives. This system excludes intentional integration of spiritual, emotional, and even physical well-being. It ignores the need for trauma-informed and healing-centered care. It is removed from land, love, and hands-on learning. It is a system that is failing many children, families, and communities.[5]

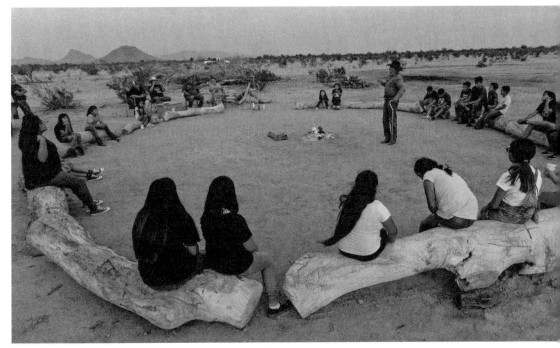

Cy Johnson (Tohono O'odham) tells stories and offers guidance to youth attendees of the annual Salt River Horse Camp, an event designed to include foster children and other youth from the tribe in traditional cultural activities.

Amidst the conversation happening in Western culture about the shortcomings of education today, we can turn to the teachings of the Indigenous educational worldview for a way forward. These precolonial systems were masterful at fostering a holistic environment that prepared every child, in an equitable way, to lead a healthy, productive, fulfilled, and happy life. In an effort to improve the health and wellness of our children today, and in an effort to give them a brighter future, we might consider finding ways to integrate an Indigenized education into all children's lives. We obviously cannot precisely mimic the social fabric of our ancestors, but we can still learn from it, draw from it, and integrate it to the best of our abilities, even if that means applying some of these strategies from home while children still attend regular public schools. We can't turn the education system on its head overnight, but we can start small, and we can start somewhere.

In our lives, we have experienced this type of education by simply spending time with our elders. Chelsey has memories of sitting at her grandparents' kitchen table for hours and hours. By watching the comings-and-goings of other relatives, by listening to conversations that adults were having, by watching them do everyday things, like cook and clean, she learned, in a subtle and indirect yet profound sense, so many valuable life lessons about how to behave, how to treat others, and what to value in life. Thosh spent endless hours shadowing spiritual leaders in his community, watching how they carried themselves humbly, how they did not waste their words, and how they led without being pushy. This time spent with elders has shaped us into who we are today, and it cannot be removed from the conversation about our wellness journeys.

From an Indigenous perspective, it is important to assume that everyone we meet has something to teach us. In this way, community is integral to our wellness because our hearts and minds remain more open at all times. Too often we walk around the world assuming ignorance on behalf of the people we come across. But when we walk around with a willingness to learn, a belief that every single person has something good to offer, and a commitment to trusting the process, we can begin to act as community once again. We can rekindle and maintain a spirit of reciprocity that is so very needed.

Remember also that it is not just other people who contribute to our education; it is the whole world around us, including plant life and animal life. Challenge yourself to learn from everyone and everything you come across. Then, observe your life begin to take on significant meaning even in small, simple moments. Observe your mind and heart constantly expanding. Be a lifelong learner, never above learning from anyone or anything.

SACRED LITTLE ONES:
INDIGENOUS PARENTING WORLDVIEW

How we parent has everything to do with the communities we foster. Traditional Indigenous parenting teaches us that in order to raise our children with a commitment to wellness and health, we must include them in every aspect of our own healthy lifestyles, we must lead by example, and we must foster a safe space for them in which these good ways of life are a normal and attainable state of being. Indigenous perspectives on parenting can help formulate this. Harsh discipline, physical abuse, yelling, and separation of child and adult social lives were all foreign concepts to Indigenous communities until Native children were forced out of their homes and into boarding schools and residential school systems. There, often at the hands of priests and nuns, they faced horrific abuses and a style of discipline previously foreign to Native communities. Precolonial Indigenous parenting, however, was loving, patient, and sweet. Here are some core tenets of traditional Indigenous parenting that many Native parents today are actively reclaiming and revitalizing.

1. *Adults can learn from children*. It is said that children's hearts are pure and that they carry teachings we forgot as we grew into adulthood. Children are not to be dismissed as ignorant or unwise—they carry a special, innocent kind of wisdom that teaches us to be better people. Today, we try to observe our

kids, to really listen to what they have to say, and to discuss and take note of the teachings in patience, compassion, and humility that come into our lives as we raise them.

2. *Every child belongs to every adult.* Children were always welcome in every home in the community; they were offered food, a place to hang out, and any comfort that they would receive in their own family's lodge. This not only kept children happy and safe, but kept parents feeling like they were not alone in the parenting journey, as is so often the case in today's world. We experienced this growing up to some extent, and this remains common practice in Native homes today. When we played with our cousins at our auntie's or uncle's house, we knew we could eat their food, take a nap, or make ourselves at home in any other way.

3. *No violence or yelling.* In Native communities, loudness, in general, tends to be viewed as obnoxious or out of place, so you can imagine that the thought of yelling at children has always been looked down upon, and the notion of violence against children, even a spanking, is unthinkable. In precolonial times, a person would have been considered less mature than a child if they could not control their temper in response to a child's tantrum or misbehavior. There was less weight on the child to act "in line" and instead more expectation on the adult to demonstrate patience and self-control.

4. *Adult social lives need not exclude children.* To this day, there are social gatherings in Native communities, like round dances and powwows, that last well into the hours of the early morning. These gatherings are always fun, like a party, but they do not have to exclude children because they are safe and alcohol-free. Western culture conditions us to think that fun can be had only without children present, which leaves adults feeling frustrated during the time they are parenting young children. We love to get a babysitter every once in a while, but it's not something that we feel we need all the time to have a thriving social life.

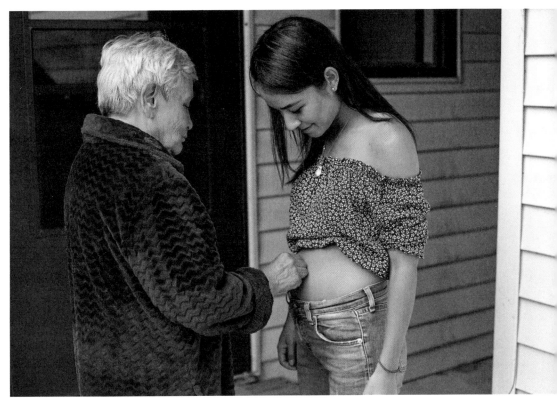

Dorothy Herman (Turtle Mountain Chippewa), Chelsey's grandma, places a needle and string on Chelsey's belly when she was nineteen weeks pregnant with her firstborn. Grandma Dorothy correctly predicted that Chelsey would have a girl.

EMBRACING AGING AND CHERISHING ELDERS

Just as we view children as sacred and beautiful, we view elders as sacred and beautiful, too. Our elders have given us so much throughout our lives. It is our honor to take care of them and to remain close to them to the end of their lives. Perhaps one of the most striking shortcomings of Western wellness culture is that it prioritizes and glorifies youth, while painting a picture of old age as being desolate and bleak. It doesn't have to be that way. In Native communities everywhere, you will see evidence of our commitment to our seniors. Tribal buildings all have elder parking. Teenagers sit with their grandparents in the bleachers at basketball games. Elders and children are served first at dinners. College students call home to their grandparents as often as they call their friends. When elders speak, we listen. When big decisions are being made, we consult those who have been on earth the longest. We never forget about them.

Always remember to spend time with your elders, to keep them included and informed, and to recognize the gift of time with them. Most important, never stop learning from them. No one can teach as profoundly and beautifully as our grandparents. They may be frail in body, but they are strong in mind and spirit, and we should always respect them and keep them close. Just remember you cannot extract elder knowledge like a sit-down interview. The only way to truly experience the mutual healing and benefits of this is to spend the time. It's just like connecting to the land. You need to spend the time. Connecting to your elders will come to be one of the most fulfilling and beautiful parts of your life. You will never regret it.

RUNNING FOR UNITY, WELLNESS, AND PEACE
THOSH

Some of my most formative experiences involved the greater O'odham community, with spiritual runs being particularly influential. In chapter 1, I talked about spiritual runs as bringing a new meaning to movement. But the spiritual runs have also affected my sense of community. As we have mentioned, you will notice a great deal of overlap and interconnection of the Seven Circles of Wellness in your life.

I miss those days when we would pile into my dad's old Suburban and drive down to the Gila River or a rural village in Tohono O'odham to attend a gathering. In 1993, we did a run that started at a place in Mexico called Ce:dagǐ Wahia (green wells) to a place called I'itoi ha Ki (home of I'itoi, a well-known medicine man in O'odham history). Once, we did a forty-four-mile relay run to honor

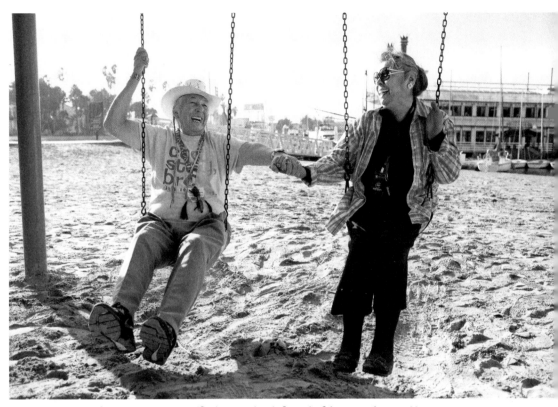

The late Charles Tailfeathers and Nancy Tailfeathers join hands for a playful moment during a Native Wellness Institute gathering.

unity, wellness, and peace in O'odham communities. Two runners at a time would run a few miles, and then another two would relieve them. This way, everyone got a chance to contribute. As we ran, we carried wooden staffs decorated with beautiful ribbons that signified various aspects of our world. We handed the staff off from one runner to the next, like an Olympic torch. We ensured that the staff, a sacred object, traveled entirely by foot from beginning to end.

I was one of the youngest kids there, riding on the back of a flatbed truck with about fifty other O'odham men to the starting point of the run. Every once in a while, people would break into our traditional songs to keep us upbeat and motivated. Others would tell jokes and make everyone laugh to mix up the energy.

It was a serious event, but it was fun. Tears, both happy and sad, were always shed at these gatherings. I loved it when families came out of their homes to watch us run by. Spectators told us that it gave them so much strength to see the men and boys running together in a ceremonial way. Most of the time, we were escorted by women and men on horseback, followed by several support vehicles. There would be stations along the way where people would quickly pass us oranges, Gatorade, or bottles of water. To see so many people standing up to honor us as we arrived gave me a strong sense of belonging and community. It made me feel like I mattered—like I belonged to something greater than myself.

Once we arrived at our destination point, we would be tired, with aching feet, and then we would have to stand for hours as elders and spiritual leaders recited long speeches about the importance of our O'odham lifeways. There was never an "agenda" or a time limit during these gatherings. It would have been very rude to interrupt and ask when it was going to end, or to leave early, so we stood patiently and paid attention. Then, the supporters from our community would come up to shake all of the runners' hands. Sometimes we'd be shaking hands with hundreds of people. Everyone would pass by, quickly expressing words of gratitude.

These are such good memories that I'll carry forever. Today, as we write this book, I am forty years old, and I continue to take part in our community runs and plan to do so as long as I can. Unfortunately, these big runs are not as prevalent today for a number of reasons. My vision is that our generations can begin to step up to keep this great tradition alive so that my daughters and all Native youth can experience how movement can strengthen not only our physical bodies, but also our ties to community, the land, our history, and our collective well-being.

As time has passed, my appreciation for these runs, and for my community, has only grown. Running is the most ancient form of movement among human beings, and it has the power to unite people from across the world who share a common purpose in the continuum of their collective life journeys. My hope for my community, and for other Indigenous communities that participate in and host spiritual runs, is that we continue this tradition and pass it on to our youth, knowing that they can carry these experiences to guide them and keep them rooted throughout life. When I see non-Indigenous communities hosting 5K runs for a cause, or marathons for charity, I am inspired and grateful that there are other cultural iterations of this important practice. I hope that youth from everywhere can find community through events that promote movement and intention in a noncompetitive, unifying way.

RETURNING TO THE REAL WORLD

As we write this book, we are in the midst of the global coronavirus pandemic. Over the past few years, we have watched devastation unfold as widespread grief and illness, coupled with the necessity to socially distance and isolate, have led to a ripple effect of health consequences. Rates of addiction, depression, and even suicide have skyrocketed. Those who have been forced to spend all day in front of computer screens to socialize, work, and learn through digital video platforms have reported feeling more alone than ever.

This has taught us a valuable lesson, one that Western society was bound to eventually learn: real-life human connection cannot be artificially replaced with technology. Community is critical. We need peer support and healthy relationships not only to live in balance, but to live at all. We must commit to actually learning and living the lessons of this pandemic. We must center, respect, and find our place in community once again, recognizing the many ways that interpersonal connection makes up the very fiber of our total well-being.

From Salt River and from Standing Rock, we both have grown up hearing the whispers and warnings of elders who have long been aware of the dangers of the internet—a modern-day trickster. One prophecy has been widely shared around Native Country over the years. It predicted that a spider web would surround the world, connecting all people like never before. The convenience and excitement that surrounded it would tempt and lure nearly everyone, but it would also bring consequences to those who became too caught in it.

Today, we have learned what those consequences are. People around the world, especially youth, are absorbed in social media, suffering from bullying, feelings of inadequacy, and divisiveness. Social media is the antithesis of Indigenous values in that it encourages individualism, arrogance, conflict, and exploitation. It creates false connection and performative persona-making rather than a true existence of quiet and humble authenticity.

When the internet first arrived not so long ago, no one could have imagined its health consequences—not only the mental health challenges, but also physical and spiritual challenges, as our online careers and schools keep us indoors, away from the land, and more sedentary than ever before. Now that we, as a global community, have observed this and experienced it, we must take steps to control and remedy it so that the next generation will not be further immersed in the artificial, emotionally starved world of technology. This should be viewed as an urgent and immediate community health need.

Rebuilding community today requires fostering our in-person connections while establishing a system of self-control and restraint in which we limit and monitor our online presence and interactions. In order to live in balance once again, we must undergo a collective return to reality, which requires a reclamation of community building. This is the only way forward. If there is one thing the pandemic and the digital generation have taught us, it is that we cannot move into the future on the trajectory of digital reliance that we have been on. If you have been living an isolated lifestyle and are not currently part of some type of identifiable community, you might wonder what community even looks like. Look no further than Native nations. Many reservations are in rural areas where internet connections and cell phone service are bad or nonexistent. Unjust as that is, there is a positive spin: our sense of real-life community has not been forgotten.

A ROCK FOR OTHERS
CHELSEY

"Hush; my little daughter must never talk about my tears"; and smiling through them, she patted my head and said, "Now let me see how fast you can run today."

—*Zitkala-Sa/Gertrude Simmons Bonnin (Yankton Sioux),*
American Indian Stories

My earliest memory is of my mom. I was two years old. We lived a short while in a B.I.A. (Bureau of Indian Affairs) housing complex on the Turtle Mountain rez, where all of the tiny identical units had chipped white paint and brightly colored window trim. My little wide feet stood on the cold speckled tiles by the bathroom doorway. I watched and waited as she cleaned the tub, preparing my nightly bath. Suddenly, unexpectedly, she screamed and jumped back. I leaned in to see what had happened. A mouse was crawling out of the drain.

I carried this memory with me for years. Finally, unsure of whether it was a figment of my imagination, I asked her whether or not it had actually happened. She laughed and said yes, it did, and that she couldn't believe I remembered. She had forgotten it herself.

I wondered why I kept that memory, and how it stayed so vivid. Eventually it dawned on me. It was the first, and one of the only, times in my life when I had ever seen anything or anyone get a rise out of my mom. She is always so calm and collected. She never shouts, screams, or makes a scene. Now that I am older and I know the story of hardship she faced during that time in her life, now that I have kids myself and better understand what it must have been like for her as a struggling young mom, I am all the more amazed by her ease.

To this day, my mom remains a steady force of strength and composure. She is a rock for so many. Me, our family, her colleagues, the students she serves, and the friends she holds dear—all know her as a pillar of reliability.

I have learned so much by watching her over the years, but rarely have I picked her brain for direct advice. When I called her on the phone recently to do just that, she was running from meeting to meeting but gladly paused to give me this: "When something bad happens, breathe, think, and try to avoid a knee-jerk reaction. Don't allow yourself to go to the worst-case scenario, because if your mind goes there, it's more likely to turn out that way. Always know that there's got to be a solution and that there will always be a better day."

Her disposition has taken her a long way; she is now a tribal college president and says that remaining "unflustered" is as important as any other part of her job. She learned how to be this way by watching her parents and grandmas over the years, seeing how they handled everything without getting bent out of shape. She said it also helped that she was given many responsibilities from a young age and has always viewed herself as capable.

In retrospect, I see how her steadiness has been such a benefit in my life, as her daughter. It grounded me and made me feel safe to explore, take risks, and walk down a fulfilling path of my own. I strive now to be a rock for others. This, to me, is the epitome of wellness. It is a trait that is not loud, attention-grabbing, or exciting. But it truly is a gift for the ones you love.

TAKE ACTION: CENTERING COMMUNITY FOR HEALTH BEYOND THE SELF

Learn

- Identify close friends, family members, communities, or groups that you are currently a part of. If you do not currently see yourself as an active part of community, consider joining a group or organization to feel more connected to those around you. Community will look different for all people—whether you are an introvert with two close friends or an extrovert with two hundred extended relatives, acknowledge those you are connected to as community.

- Identify your role in this community. Ask yourself, What are my gifts, what can I offer, and how can I contribute?
- Remember that community is something you can *build*. Seek people who are of the same mindset, on a similar journey of wellness, and carry similar values and with whom you can be mutually supportive.
- Talk to your family members: spouse, parents, children, extended relatives. State your intention to build and maintain a strong bond and connection with them. Ask them about their thoughts on this as well.
- As you step into your wellness journey, examine these questions: Who are the leaders of my family? And how do I support them, knowing that eventually I may step in to fill their position as a pillar for my network?
- Observe how leaders in your family, clan, and community speak, pray, and respond to things. Begin to recognize the traits they carry, and set a goal of learning to embody those qualities.
- Expand your definition of "relative" and recognize the ways that your actions and behavior impact plant life, animal life, and the world beyond you.

Engage

- Put yourself out there. Start showing up at meetings, events, and gatherings that your community is hosting. Remember to smile and greet people (with whatever greeting suits the cultural context), and to teach your children to do the same.
- At community gatherings, always offer to help however you can—set up and take down, arrange chairs, prepare or serve food, donate money and supplies. Remember that any form of giving is a commitment to community and is always appreciated by the group.
- Initiate a family meeting or talking circle on a regular basis to set aside time for intentional conversation with your family. Ensure that everyone gets a chance to speak and that everyone who is present is actively listening to the speaker.

Do not set a time limit. Let people talk and be heard. This should happen frequently in the home, approximately once a month.

- Find a mentor for career, traditional teachings, or whatever your focus may be, and respectfully ask whether that person is willing to guide you. Focus on spending time with your mentor and observing, on their own time, rather than asking questions to "take" information too quickly.

- Invite others to join you in any activities that have to do with your wellness: cooking, planting, movement, art, spending time outdoors, etc. Be mindful of building community around health-oriented activities.

Optimize

- You are a contributing member of your community. You are participating, present, and involved, and so are your loved ones and children.

- You are in good communication and good standing with your family. You are a compassionate, careful listener who offers a safe space for others.

- Over time, you have observed the ways that your efforts toward good health have positively influenced those around you, and people have thanked you for being a good role model or an inspiration for them and their loved ones.

- People call on you to guide them, to advise them, to mentor them, and to assist them. When you are not present, people feel your absence.

- You are always mindful of gratitude for your ancestors and hope for the future, recognizing that community transcends time and space and is intergenerational.

INTERSECTION WITH OTHER CIRCLES

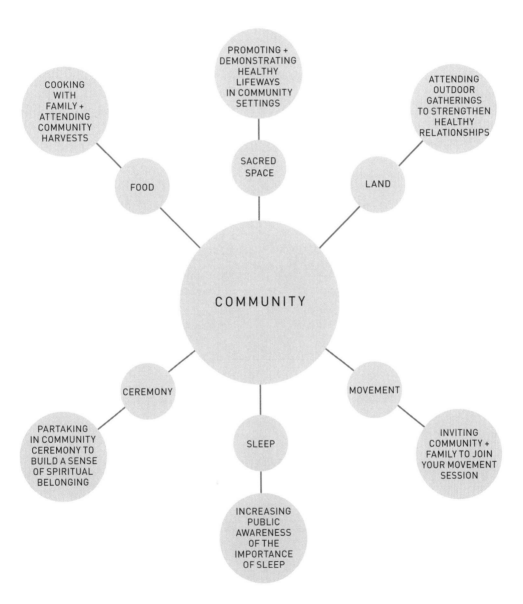

COOKING WITH FAMILY + ATTENDING COMMUNITY HARVESTS

PROMOTING + DEMONSTRATING HEALTHY LIFEWAYS IN COMMUNITY SETTINGS

ATTENDING OUTDOOR GATHERINGS TO STRENGTHEN HEALTHY RELATIONSHIPS

FOOD

SACRED SPACE

LAND

COMMUNITY

CEREMONY

SLEEP

MOVEMENT

PARTAKING IN COMMUNITY CEREMONY TO BUILD A SENSE OF SPIRITUAL BELONGING

INCREASING PUBLIC AWARENESS OF THE IMPORTANCE OF SLEEP

INVITING COMMUNITY + FAMILY TO JOIN YOUR MOVEMENT SESSION

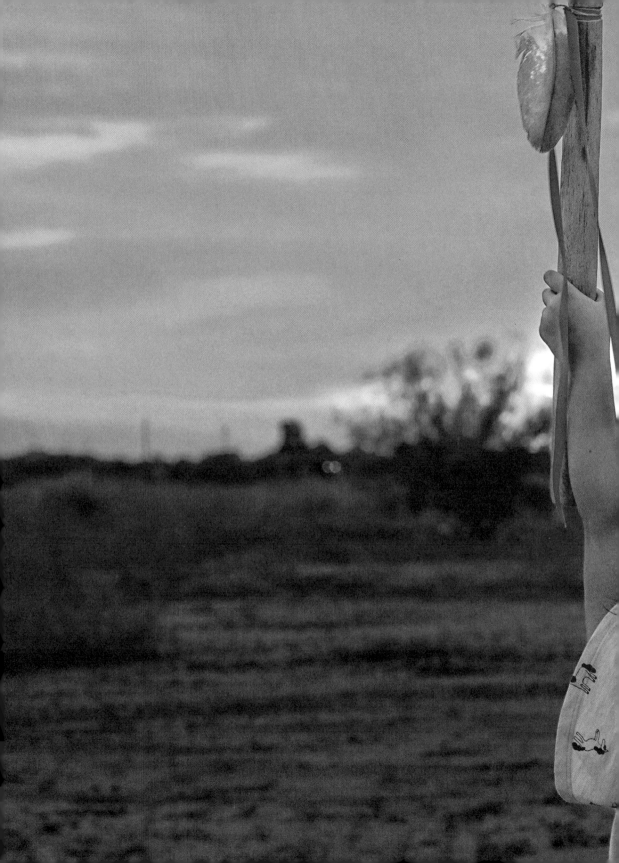

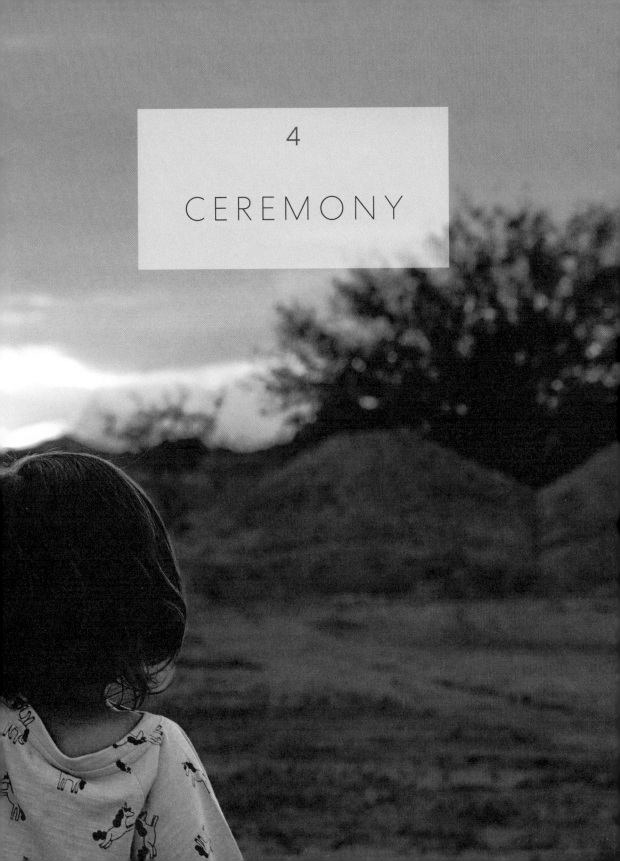

4

CEREMONY

We are only human, and all of our rituals reflect that . . . There is no mystery in it at all.

—*Albert White Hat (Sicangu Lakota),* Life's Journey—Zuya:
Oral Teachings from Rosebud

ACCEPTING THE STORMS OF LIFE
CHELSEY

After a morning swimming at our favorite spot at the river, we piled into the truck to head out before the desert heat reached its peak. We didn't feel ready to go home to accept the day's end, so we went for a cruise around the rez. Alo wanted to see her grandpa Tony, so we pulled up to his house and tapped the horn. He walked toward us through his front lawn, followed by Cowboy, Sko'mag, Bandit, and the rest of his happy pack of dogs. Instead of going inside to visit, we stayed in the truck so baby Westyn could stay asleep in her car seat. Tony leaned on the edge of the passenger side window and started to tell us about his day. In the middle of his story, out of nowhere and quite suddenly, a whirlwind came billowing toward us.

If you're not familiar with whirlwinds (weather phenomena that are essentially miniature tornadoes), life in the desert will introduce you. They are fairly common, and they range in size from a few inches in diameter to something that could envelop a house. This one was at least as big as our Nissan Titan. Not having grown up with them myself, I watched in awe as it came toward us at full speed. Thosh said, "Jump in, Dad!" Tony replied, "I'm fine, just cover the girls."

Previous page: In honor of the National Day for Truth and Reconciliation, also known as Orange Shirt Day, Alo Collins (Anishinaabe, Lakota, O'odham, Osage, and Seneca-Cayuga), age four, holds a prayer staff toward the setting sun. The orange ribbon and eagle plume tied to the staff represent the children—both survivors and those who never made it home—who were once forced to attend abusive educational institutions in Canada.

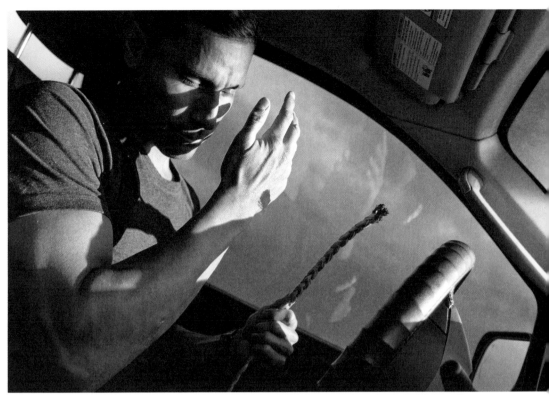

While pulled over on the side of the highway on a road trip, Thosh smudges with sweetgrass and offers a family prayer for safe travels.

We rolled up the windows while Tony glanced over his shoulder to evaluate the approaching vortex. His calm demeanor made it evident that he had seen hundreds of these over the course of his life in Arizona. As it came nearer, he turned his back to it and casually lowered his camouflage bucket hat over his eyes. A moment later, we were enveloped in a gray mass. I couldn't believe how quickly the scene went from sunshine to darkness. The sound of the gusty wind harmonized with the ping-pang of rocks and twigs that peppered the outside of the truck.

Then, just as suddenly as it had come, the whirlwind disappeared across the road, leaving hardly a trace behind. Our daughters remained relaxed, blissfully unaware of the weather event. I felt relieved that we were able to get the windows up in time to shield them from the debris. I thought, If only we could always protect them from all of the storms they will face in life.

We rolled down the windows again to the sound of Tony's laughter as he brushed himself off. He seemed to almost enjoy the harsh elemental greeting, like a playful tackle from an older brother.

On second thought, I realized, I hope that our girls will learn to face challenges the way that their grandpa handled the whirlwind: calmly, with bravery and a little bit of humor. That would be better than shielding them from everything.

Hardship is inevitable. This is why we always say that wellness is about balance, not about perfection. It is about getting through life's journey, not arriving at an end goal. We make mistakes and we learn from them. We hurt, and then we heal. To be well is not to avoid bad times; it is to keep a set of tools that will help us face challenges without being completely thrown off. Sometimes, the idea of well-being is conflated with "total happiness" and is taught with a "pull yourself up by your bootstraps" mentality. But that approach is neither responsible nor honest. Tragedies will strike. Days will be bad. No one is a lesser person for not being able to control or avoid these basic human realities.

We have seen our parents, our grandparents, our mentors, our cultural leaders, and countless other people exemplify these traits of peacefulness, grit, compassion, and resilience. We have seen it on a micro scale, in personal situations, where time and time again, our people emerge from the most traumatic of experiences and remain not only functional but incredibly kindhearted and giving. We have seen it on a macro scale, in community, where Indigenous nations have remained intact and empowered, committed to sovereignty, to continuity of culture, and to standing up for the earth, the youth, and the water, despite facing constant resistance. We are so proud of our people and the strength that they exemplify. How do they do it? The answer is complex, but at the center of it remains one key component: *ceremony*.

Ceremony has always been a hallmark of Indigenous culture, and it still is. Right now, as the world is in the midst of a heightened state of chaos and intensity, ceremony is more important than ever. The severity of the climate crisis is perhaps the most profound manifestation of a world out of balance, caused largely by a human population devoid of the instinct to reciprocate. Natural disasters are intensifying, health problems are surging, politics are polarizing, and as the environment suffers, millions of people are suffering too. In an out-of-balance world, according to Takelma Siletz elder Agnes Baker Pilgrim, "ritual and ceremony create the energy of reciprocity."[1]

Ceremony has carried Indigenous people through what has seemed like insurmountable circumstances. And it continues to carry us through this era of healing. Life today is challenging. We have the highest rates of health disparities, our languages and lands have been stolen from us, we have experienced abuse, we have survived genocide, and now we are attempting to recover from economic deprivation. And yet, we are here, we are moving forward, and in many cases we are deeply fulfilled by our culture, which urges us to always find the deeper, spiritual purpose in each day. It is quite remarkable to witness Indigenous resilience. This perhaps can serve as a point of hope and inspiration for everyone.

Our elders teach us that there is always an opportunity to return to balance. When we do this, not only can we survive, but we can thrive. *Ceremony* is the system of knowledge and the balancing force that works to anchor and call back this balance. The concept of ceremony, and how to incorporate it into one's life, will be different for everyone. Perhaps you are an Indigenous person who attends and contributes to the private and personal ceremonies that come from your own community and family. Or perhaps you are a person who has learned rituals, religions, prayers, or other modalities of finding peacefulness. These all fit within the circle of ceremony. No matter who you are, you may learn how to *walk in a ceremonial way* or *live each day like a ceremony*, which means to carry yourself with compassion, dignity, respect, honor, and humility.

This book invites all readers to understand what it means to respect Indigenous culture while learning from our ways of life. So it is with love and concern for the safety and privacy of our own communities that we kindly remind all readers that there are modes of spirituality, ceremony, ritual, mindfulness, and other relevant practices that are true to *you* and can be found in your own meaningful way. Indigenous spirituality and ceremonies should never be mocked, mimicked, or copied. Later in the chapter, we delve into the history of Indigenous religious suppression, spiritual discrimination, and the harms of Indigenous cultural appropriation in the modern wellness industry. These are critical pieces of this conversation that anyone embarking on a journey of spiritual discovery should learn. According to journalist Greg Tate, "appropriation and the fetishizing of cultures . . . alienates those whose culture is being appropriated."[2]

One of the beautiful things about Indigenous culture is that we do not feel the need to convert others or to persuade anyone that our type of spirituality is the best or most righteous way. If you already follow a spiritual or religious tradition, we encourage you to keep doing so. We encourage you to dig into the ancient and ongoing chains of knowledge that come from your own nationality, heritage, and family history and to incorporate those methods and teachings into your life today. If that knowledge has been lost, you can find it again, and the journey can be deeply healing for you. Not only will cultivating an authentic spiritual or ritualistic practice be the best way to avoid cultural appropriation, it will also be the most sustainable and true. Simply put, it will feel right. If something feels awkward or performative, you are less likely to stick with it. Authenticity is both more respectful and more effective for everyone.

Learning how to transform or elevate one or more aspects of your everyday routine into ritual is perhaps the best way to bring ceremony into your life. In this way, events that would be otherwise mundane become significant, symbolic, and meaningful. Esther Perel, a psychotherapist and relationships expert, says that "routines get us through the day, while rituals guide us through life."[3] So whether you incorporate words of gratitude at family mealtime, go outside to greet the sun as it rises, breathe mindfully, give thanks for land and water when you spend time outdoors, ritualistically apply your skincare, exercise with an intention for community wellness, light a special candle at the same time each night as you cozy up to a book, or create a special good-night routine with your spouse and children—let your mode of ceremony and ritual bring you peace, grounding, healing, enlightenment, and always the courage to move forward steadily.

HOW CEREMONY HEALS
⊕ Ceremony Medicine Wheel ⊕

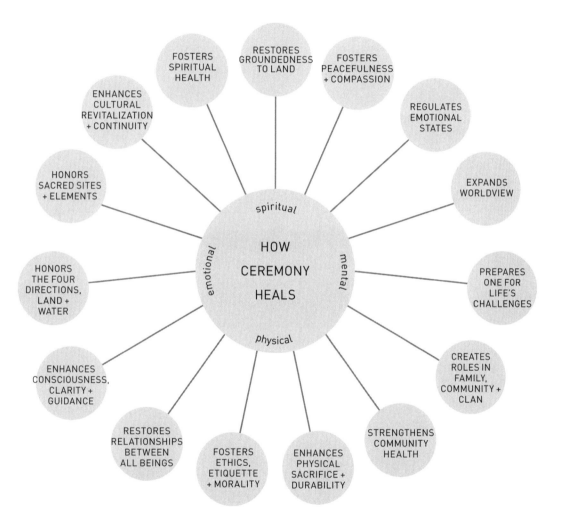

SPIRITUAL

Today, we live in a spiritually repressed society, but all people can learn to walk in a ceremonial way, to reclaim ritual, and to utilize mindfulness to heighten awareness and bring peace, leading to a more grounded, grateful, and whole existence.

EMOTIONAL

People who are anchored in spirituality are resilient—able to weather the storms that life inevitably brings. A mindfulness or peacefulness practice, like meditation or ritual, will help us learn to accept the balance of good and bad that life will bring. When we remain grateful for what we have, even when we experience loss, we are able to maintain emotional stability throughout the highs and lows that come our way.

MENTAL

Incorporating rituals throughout the day, and practicing those rituals consistently at the same time every day, is one way to open up mental space for the demands of our careers and the logistical side of life, rather than being constantly bombarded by noise. We may use ceremony or ritual to carve a path of clarity in the mind.

PHYSICAL

When we incorporate prayer or set intentions for healing, prosperity, and wellness as we move our bodies and exert ourselves physically, we build strength from the inside out: starting with our inner spirit, moving into the body, and then exerting outward through our energy.

UNDERSTANDING INDIGENOUS CEREMONIES

From time immemorial, in every Indigenous nation, ceremony has been an integral aspect of healing and well-being, serving functional purposes in everyday life, like bringing guidance, clarity, and values, while also serving higher purposes for the world at large, like bringing balance and peace and maintaining a human relationship to the earth and the elements. There is no universal Native American religion, and indeed there are no two Native families who practice spirituality or prayer in exactly the same way. We do not have guidelines written down in a holy book, nor do we maintain a pan-Indian set of beliefs. The absence of a written or bureaucratized organization should not be confused with a lack of structure or intention. The oral tradition and careful transference of knowledge through familial and clan lineages has worked to keep protocol, guidelines, and intricate systems of ceremonial knowledge in place, which in turn keep communities functioning not just spiritually but also politically, economically, and in many other ways.

As time has passed over millennia, many ceremonies have remained largely unchanged, but they have not become antiquated. Rather, like any other discipline that becomes studied more and more, spiritual knowledge builds upon itself, grows, and becomes more robust. The teachings that ceremony and ritual carry have remained remarkably relevant through the ebbs and flows of history, designed by divine genius to answer the ever-changing needs of the land and people.

Sometimes ceremonies are individual (a daily prayer with smudging), and other times they involve an entire community (a Sun Dance). Some ceremonies happen in small groups (a sweat lodge), and others are for a family to commemorate milestones (a coming of age). Some are an annual display of reverence that serves economic functions (such as a planting or harvesting ceremony), and others honor the life-giving forces of the universe (like the rain or sun). Some ceremonies have been direct responses to community tragedy (such as the Ghost Dance), and others respond to personal tragedy (a wiping of the tears). Some are direct responses to emerging community needs (such as reburying remains of ancestors that have been uncovered at construction sites) or environmental emergencies (praying to stop an oil pipeline). Some ceremonies take place in one location and require solitude and self-confinement (such as vision seeking), and others are group journeys that traverse the land (such as a spiritual run). Some Indigenous ceremonies uniquely celebrate the same things that other cultures often celebrate (like weddings), and others are a means for Native families to express special reverence for moments that they deem sacred (such as a baby's first food or laugh).

All ceremonies are a renewal of relationships between people, the natural world, and elemental forces. All ceremonies are opportunities to rekindle the goodness in

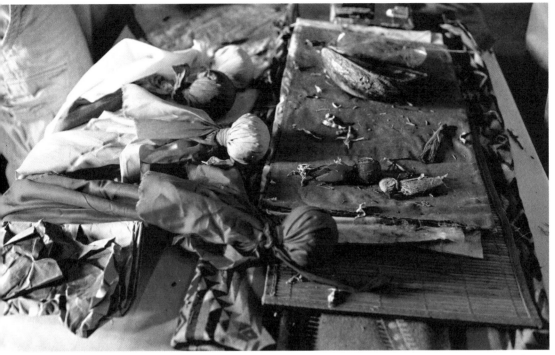

Medicine bundles placed on a table at a Native Wellness Institute gathering. Participants were invited to make their own medicine ties, a bundle of prayers, so that they could carry the good energy of the gathering with them wherever they went. This ceremony was gifted to the Native Wellness Institute by Charles Tailfeathers, a Cree elder.

humanity by showing respect to the nonhuman entities that keep us alive. All ceremonies are ways for participants to learn how to live honorably and to walk with dignity. In ceremony, we actively seek guidance from Creator in hopes of learning to be stronger, more giving, more balanced people. Because of the sacrifices and hardships involved in ceremony, we are reminded of our weaknesses and we are grounded in our humility, an ancestral value that is held in high regard.

In most cases, ceremonies are conducted or overseen by medicine people, elders, and community leaders who have grown up engrained in the culture that surrounds the ceremonies. Knowledge to lead and participate in Indigenous ceremonies requires cultural context. Our medicine people have spent their lives learning, studying, practicing, giving, and inheriting knowledge that has been passed down in their families for centuries. It is a highly specialized form of medicine that cannot be learned from a book, a workshop, or in school and most certainly cannot be co-opted or practiced by someone who was raised outside of the culture. These ceremonial leaders and medicine people do not perform, publicize, or show off their gifts. They do not even charge money for their services (although it is considered polite to offer to them what you can if they have helped you).

In Indigenous communities, ceremonies are usually private and not open to the public or advertised. These are grassroots gatherings with no big funding sources and certainly no registration fees, so participants always give and contribute what they can in the form of food, labor, or other needed resources. Photography, documentation, and reporting are typically not allowed. These gatherings are sacred, and cultural privacy is highly valued. Medicine people do not seek glory or fame in any way. If a person wants to share stories about ceremony, they do so with select people, on an as-needed basis, with discretion and care. If a person goes around bragging or saying too much about things that they saw or experienced, they are held accountable by their community.

Ceremonies are held dear to our communities as precious healing tools and opportunities for community gathering that we cannot live without. Ceremony is not a luxury retreat or a performance for our people—it is a lifeline. This is why we avoid exploitation at all costs.

Indigenous relatives, we can't tell you anything new about how important ceremonies are—you know this. We simply hope to encourage you to keep participating in and prioritizing these gatherings, despite any discrimination or barriers that you may face. We hope that you find a way to pass these on to your children, recognizing how such practices can shape and nurture their total well-being. Ceremony is health care, it is community care, and it is something that you deeply deserve.

The Science of Ceremony

For centuries, outsiders have discriminated against Indigenous spirituality by either demonizing it (Christian missionaries conflated it with devil worship) or dismissing it as primitive superstition. Dr. Michael Yellow Bird is dean and professor, Faculty of Social Work, at the University of Manitoba, and an Indigenous studies and social work scholar who is a member of the Three Affiliated Tribes: the Mandan, Hidatsa, and Arikara in North Dakota. A portion of his work focuses on the science and impact of ceremony and spirituality and the robust evidence that supports what Native people have always known: that ceremonies, both secular and spiritual, play an important role in contributing to health and well-being and can heal us in ways that other things, such as diet and exercise, simply cannot.

Dr. Yellow Bird has utilized genetic research, evolutionary biology and psychology, history, traditional narratives, exercise science, biochemistry, contemplative science, and neuroscience to demonstrate the positive, healing effects of Indigenous healing methodologies. When we dance, sing, run, speak, and pray in our languages; sleep well; recount traditional stories; learn from and spend time on the land; gather in community; move with intention; eat with gratitude; and sit in contemplation as our ancestors did (and, most important, when we do these consistently), a number of remarkable things take place: we rebuild our mitochondria, known as "powerhouses" of the cells inside us, that produce the energy needed by our cells to power our heart, liver, muscles, and brain. We trigger neurogenesis, the growth of new neurons in the brain that play an important role in neural plasticity, preserve cognitive function, and repair damaged brain cells. Moreover, we protect our brains against depression, anxiety, suicidal ideation, and stress; we raise the levels of important brain chemicals such as serotonin and dopamine, which contribute to feelings of happiness and pleasure; and we activate the left side of our brain's prefrontal cortex, the part of our brain associated with feelings of happiness, joy, optimism, and well-being. In every sense of the word, we are practicing wellness, and we are healing.[4]

In short, the healing properties of ceremony, spirituality, and of a ceremonial life are real and have tangible, positive consequences for health and health care.

The Power of Silence

Our ancestors have always valued silence, and many in our communities continue the practice of actively seeking silence. Many Indigenous nations have been practicing specific isolation ceremonies for thousands of years, in which people go off by themselves for days without contacting others so that they can hear and receive teachings without the disturbance or influence of other humans. In ancestral times, silence was also valued greatly as a part of daily life and etiquette. Many elders have shared with us that they miss the days when people were comfortable with silence and careful with their words. In those days, they say, the sixth sense, or a sense of intuition and gut instinct, was stronger. In any case, quiet time for self-reflection, learning from the natural world, and seeking visions was always recognized as an important step in intellectual and spiritual growth.

Today, the world is noisier than ever, so the ancestral practice of seeking silence may be an even more critical health practice than it has been before. Noise, after all, isn't just an annoying disturbance. Its presence can lead to serious health consequences. Studies show that prolonged exposure to noise can lead to heart disease, heart attacks, high blood pressure, strokes, diabetes, dementia, and depression. White noise, or background noise, has also been shown to make people act more aggressively.[5]

You can incorporate silence into your life in a number of ways: literally (voices off), digitally (devices off), by avoiding crowds and chaos, or by creating visual silence (turning off TVs and lights; closing your eyes). Taking intentional time for quiet is necessary. Some also seek silence through very specific learned practices, like meditation, while others have developed more personalized, intuitive mindfulness and quieting techniques. However silence is sought, such practices are an important piece of personal wellness and health care that many of us are missing from our lives today.

To begin your silence-seeking practice, we recommend growing accustomed to silence in moments when you typically add noise to your environment as a crutch. For example, while waiting in line or for a ride, avoid looking at your phone and its "visual noise." Instead, observe the world around you. Make this a habit, and see how long it takes you to become comfortable *not* looking at an electronic device. You can also incorporate silence when you are in your car. Typically, people turn on a podcast or music right away. Try going an entire week where you remain silent and undistracted rather than listening to some-thing through the speakers while on the road. Finally, try moving in silence. Just as with driving, music and podcasts tend to go hand-in-hand with exercise these days. Observe how much more intentional your thoughts can be as you move without anything playing. Let your waiting time, your driving time, and your movement practice become ceremonial through more silence.

MINDFUL MILESTONES AND SACRED CELEBRATIONS

In the realm of ceremony are the big moments in life that we all love to celebrate—weddings, holidays, a new year, and so on. A shared trait of cultures worldwide is to take time to acknowledge these moments through singing, dancing, per-forming rituals, praying, and setting renewed intentions. We love to learn about the way that different people from different cultures celebrate different moments, and we have found that there is no end to traditions that have remained steadfastly focused on the prayerful, mindful intention of these special times.

Part of our wellness journey in our home has been the return to mindful mile-stones and sacred celebrations. We have noticed that some popular American holidays, like Christmas or Valentine's Day, tend to bring stress or sadness when the emphasis is placed too heavily on the commercial aspect of the holiday and not enough on its deeper meaning. Don't lose sight of the deeper meaning of whatever holidays or milestones you share with your family. These events should not stretch family finances or cause us to be overly concerned with image and ap-pearance. That takes the heart out of them. They should always be times to focus on family, food, and spirit.

We love to share the story of our intertribal wedding. Our three-day celebra-tion was focused on setting intentions for our shared life and future together, but it was equally focused on bringing together our families and friends in a spiritual way. Most of it took place outdoors, so we did not have to stress about spending

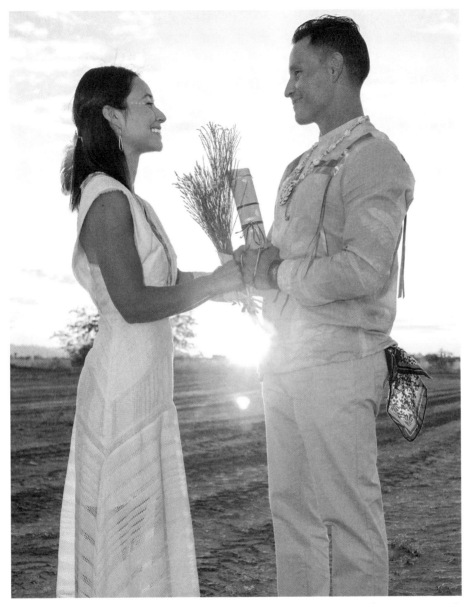

At sunset, just after their wedding ceremony, Chelsey and Thosh hold an ironwood staff, the strongest wood found in the desert, to symbolize their shared intention to uphold a strong, safe, and nurturing relationship. During the ceremony, their family and friends joined them in sharing a commitment to this intention.

thousands of dollars on a fancy venue. We bought simple, inexpensive clothes that our moms and aunties turned into stunning regalia with their beadwork and sewing. We were honored by the presence of our loved ones and relatives from all over the world—people from many walks of life and different cultures. They came together in ceremony with us, and with medicine ties, we all agreed to pray not only for a solid future for our family, but that all of the people with us there would move forward with a good heart and mind to be a part of the sacred circle of all who were in attendance.

We have also decolonized the way that we understand the New Year. Instead of celebrating the date set on the Gregorian calendar, because that is not something our ancestors celebrated, we host a big dinner with Indigenous foods on the winter and summer solstices, acknowledging the earth's natural renewals and the changing seasons of life. We have also created a family "winter count," which means that we keep a big piece of muslin fabric that we take out only once a year. Then we decide as a family what we will draw on it—each year one small symbol to represent what came to pass that was special in our family that year. This will be a cherished item to pass down through the generations.

Whatever culture you come from, and whatever milestones or moments are important to you, remember to emphasize connection and to focus less on the commercial. This transforms holidays from being a potentially stressful time to being true celebrations that contribute to our overall well-being once again.

EVERYDAY CEREMONY: TURNING ROUTINE INTO RITUAL

Incorporating ceremony into your life might sound lofty or confusing, especially if it isn't a concept that you grew up with. Or even if you have grown up attending tribal ceremonies, you might not be sure how to incorporate other types of ceremony into your day-to-day wellness routine. The answer is *ritual*. One of the easiest, most natural ways to bring ceremony into your everyday life is to consciously turn one or more of your routines into ritual. Remember, routines are good because they provide structure and order, but rituals add creativity, intention, and even vulnerability into our lives.[6] In short, they add a deeper sense of meaning and purpose. Here are two scenarios, one in an individual context and one in a group context, of what this could look like.

Scenario 1—Waking-Up Routine vs. Waking-Up Ritual: A common *waking-up routine* includes abruptly waking up to a loud smartphone alarm, picking up said smartphone, scrolling for a few minutes or checking email, then rushing to get ready and out the door. Most who do this routine are simply trying to be hardworking and efficient, and there is nothing wrong with that. However, it can be harmful to turn our minds toward "tasks" first thing in the morning, as this breeds anxiety and stress over time. Instead, try making mornings a ritual.

A *waking-up ritual* can be different. Use an alarm clock, not your phone, to wake you (try an old-school digital or analog clock, or a wake-up light that mimics the sunrise). Then, sit up in bed and take deep breaths—we recommend seven breaths to acknowledge the four cardinal directions along with above, below, and all-around. Deep inhaling and exhaling right away in the morning can decrease anxiety.[7] As you breathe, think about something you are grateful for, and let this thought bring a smile to your face. Next, do something creative right away. For instance, keep a notepad on your nightstand and write down what you remember about your dreams. Or draw a picture of something you hope to see or do today. Now you are ready to get out of bed with a whole new perspective, viewing the day as an opportunity, not a task.

Scenario 2—Dinner Routine vs. Dinner Ritual: Many people already have a *dinner routine* in which their family gathers at the same time every night to eat dinner, and the conversation leads where it may. There is nothing wrong with a dinner routine, but it can begin to feel mundane and chore-like if deeper meaning is not consciously brought to the table. Try turning this routine into a ritual at least once a week.

A *dinner ritual* can look like this: Appoint each person to a special task, like setting the table. Kids especially enjoy feeling helpful. Before eating, ask one person to offer a "giving of thanks," which doesn't necessarily need to be viewed in a religious context—simply a verbal act of reverence for all of the plants, animals, and people who made the meal happen and for those who are present. Make sure that no TV, phones, or other electronic devices are making noises in the background. This way, conversation is centered. Next, use a conversation prompt. Go around the table and ask everyone to say one thing that they are grateful for, or one thing that they learned that day. If it's a special meal, like a birthday, ask each person to share a favorite memory about the person who is being celebrated.

There are countless other moments throughout your day when you can transform routine into ritual, including but not limited to

- Applying skincare products and cosmetics
- Getting dressed and picking out clothes with careful intention
- Taking an intentionally cleansing shower or bath
- Having a regular artistic project, such as painting, playing music, or writing
- Cooking with deeper intention
- Making morning coffee or evening tea
- Having nighttime rituals with children or spouse

HOW I BECAME "SUN"
THOSH

Once in a while my mom and dad will tell my birth story and how I got my name, Thosh, which is also spelled T-a-s, meaning "day" or "sun," depending on how it's being used in the O'odham language. They tell how my mom was having a hard time with labor giving birth to me. She chose to have a home birth, and at the time my parents lived in town just down the street from the rez. My dad decided to call his friend Norman for advice on what to do. Norman, a Yavapai man from the Fort McDowell rez near our community, was a spiritual leader within the Native American Church community. He advised my dad to get some of the plant medicine, wet it, and then dry it in the sun and pray to it, asking the medicine and sun rays to help with the birthing process. So that's what my dad did, and finally I was born. Since my parents used the sun to help, they decided to call me Tas.

I didn't hear this story until I was about fifteen years old, and when I heard it I felt more of a connection to my name. Until then, I just knew the name had to do with the sun and that the sun was special to our people. But when I heard the story, I felt proud. I felt that the sun rays were a part of my medicine and that from that time on I should be using the rays to help me in my life journey.

Not only was I proud that the sun played a specific role in my name from birth, but I felt empowered that I was brought into the world in a ceremonial way. Knowing there was conscious spiritual intention behind the decisions of my parents during my birth process brought a warm sense of belonging to me. I knew that I was meant to be in this world and that soon I would discover my purpose here. I believe this has been a part of the foundation of my upbringing.

I have a few items that were made for me while I was in my mom's womb. One is a beaded bracelet that Norman's wife made. My mom gave it to me when I graduated from high school; she'd been keeping it all through my childhood. She brought it out and told me, "Norman's wife made this for you before you were born; she said to give it to you when turned eighteen or so." I was so surprised to receive it, mainly because of how long my mom had kept it before she presented it to me. I also liked how the beaded design on it looked like something you would have seen on someone's beaded regalia from the early 1980s. Once again, I felt so empowered and loved that someone who had not yet met me decided to make a gift for me to be presented to me as a young adult.

Another item made for me at birth was my cradleboard. Just knowing that I spent time in one during my sacred years of development brings to me a sense of belonging—belonging to a continuation of our Indigeneity. It makes me feel comforted and empowered that everything was done with the intention of restoring our Indigeneity. For myself as a parent, this is some of the basis of my understanding of what conscious Indigenous parenting is.

These small gifts and the stories that go with them have played a critical role in my Indigenous self-actualization. I want my daughters to have these experiences and more. I want many more children in the future to have this life experience where every aspect of their upbringing is done with ceremonial intention so that they too can feel this warm sense of love, belonging, and purpose.

WITNESSING WHOLENESS
CHELSEY

I grew up going to a Sun Dance ceremony in the Black Hills each summer with my dad. We would start the journey in Fort Yates, on our ranch on the Standing Rock Reservation, where we lived. We'd pack up the truck with camping gear and then drive south for eight hours through the other reservations of the Great Sioux Nation, passing through towns like Wakpala, where my grandma Thelma grew up; then Eagle Butte, where we'd stop at Taco John's. Finally, after a long westward stretch on the interstate in South Dakota, we'd make it to Spearfish, an old mining town at the foot of the Black Hills. There, my dad would stop at a grocery store to load up the truck with about a hundred pounds of meat. This would be his contribution to the communal cook shack at our camp, which would be our home for the next week or so.

I admit that I did not particularly look forward to going to ceremony. It was a long drive, it was a lot of preparation, and it was a lot of work once we got there. It took me away from friends, technology, and other adolescent comforts. But I always felt glad once we arrived, and by the time we left, I felt renewed and fulfilled, never regretting one single moment of it. It would be these days at ceremony that would anchor my wellness journey for the rest of my life.

The week at Sun Dance began the moment you entered the Black Hills—a powerful, ever-shifting place that for me acted as a portal to somewhere entirely different from the rest of the world. We saw all four seasons in a matter of days. From the blistering one-hundred-degree heat of noon to a dusting of hail at 4 a.m. to a relentless downpouring thunderstorm—we felt it all. It was vivid and intense and tough, and it made me understand why my people have always viewed the Black Hills as a sacred place. It is as if the elements showed up in their mightiest forms to remind us how to pray, to let us feel tough love, and to demonstrate solidarity with our sacrifice. By showing their power, they taunted us to pray harder.

As a kid, I enjoyed the fact that even though ceremony was such a serious event with protocols to learn and follow, none of it felt forced or scary. In fact, it seemed like the more important or revered an adult, the kinder and more easygoing that adult was. I will never forget the feeling of sitting at the feet of my elders, who sat in front of their tents on their lawn chairs, smiling and taking in visitors. My dad taught me to take tobacco to them as an offering, which is a sign of respect in Lakota culture, and in exchange they would tell me stories. Their eyes and smiles were soft and made me feel right at home.

All of them were our grandmas and grandpas, just as all of the other adults at the camp were our aunties and uncles, even though most of us were not related by blood. Our traditional kinship structures came alive during Sun Dance, as did our traditional values. No one drank alcohol, posed for photographs, or used foul language. We all woke up before the sunrise and went to sleep with the sunset. We shared food, laughter, duties, and above all, prayers. By contrast to a lot of the hardships we experienced during day-to-day life on our reservations, this was an opportunity to see our community functioning in its original truth, power, and wholeness.

Out of respect for my community, I won't go into any more detail about what a Sun Dance entails. I will say, however, that nothing else I've ever seen, witnessed, or participated in made such an impact on me. It was hard, but it was all good. I now realize that it was a holistic education. In such a short period of time, I learned big life lessons that I never would have figured out in school or any other setting. It made me understand how to be grateful, how to respect life, the importance of sacrifice, the gift of community, and the meaning of honor and reverence.

When I think about how formative and character-building those experiences were for me as a youth, and then I think about how all of my ancestors in precolonial times grew up with that type of education on a much more regular basis, I begin to grasp an iota of an understanding of not only their grit, but their level of sheer spiritual enlightenment and overall peacefulness. While many people in today's capitalist society are striving for wealth in the form of manufactured material goods and money, I pray that my children can live closer to a ceremonial way.

WHEN WE WEREN'T ALLOWED TO BE, AND OUR NEW ERA OF RECLAMATION

We often ponder the thought that spiritual health and ceremonial knowing for all people on these lands could have been thriving today if only Indigenous beliefs and ideas hadn't been actively shut down for so long. Evidence shows that Indigenous people were ready, in many ways, to *exchange* culture with settlers and missionaries—that's why our ancestors helped and took care of these newcomers—and they also were open to hearing about Christianity and other new ideas. But the Europeans had no interest in exchanging or learning from our worldview—only taking and repressing. And one of the things they took from our ancestors was the freedom to practice spirituality. The church and the government worked hand in hand in their mission to "kill the Indian and save the man."[8] During this era, Native children from every nation were stolen from their homes and communities and forced to attend abusive, assimilative institutions called boarding schools in the United States and residential schools in Canada. Countless children died in these schools. In 2021 alone, the remains of thousands of Indigenous children as young as age three were found in unmarked graves at these school sites.

In the 1800s, the federal government aimed to systemically stamp out Native American culture and religion. The Bureau of Indian Affairs enacted the 1883

Indian Religious Crimes Code, a system which gave Indian agents on Reservations the authority to ban medicine men from practicing and to restrict Native people from holding ceremonies and sacred dances, which they deemed heathenistic. Many people today are shocked to find out that this legislation was not repealed until 1978, with the passing of the American Indian Religious Freedom Act. Before that, untold thousands of Native people faced harsh punishments, like ration withholding and imprisonment, because of their attempts to continue their cultural practices.[9] During this era, some Native people who resisted religious suppression ultimately faced the punishment of death. Notably, in 1889, between 250 and 300 innocent Mniconjou Lakota were massacred by the United States Army at Wounded Knee because the Army felt threatened by their participation in the Ghost Dance.[10]

Indigenous communities continue to reel from the traumatic effects of spiritual repression. Many Native people today still do not have the freedom to practice ceremonies and Indigenous spirituality because they have been violently removed and disconnected from their communities through systems that have sought to tear Indigenous families and nations apart, whether through residential schools or a racist child welfare system. Given centuries of spiritual suppression, and then the hard work of overcoming discrimination and reclaiming these practices, you can understand why Indigenous people today are often quite protective of their ceremonies. We are still holding on to them closely and tightly because we know what it's like to have them taken away from us.

The first task for non-Indigenous readers on their path to a wellness practice inspired by Indigenous ideas is education. Many people simply do not know that their attempts to adapt Native rituals are harmful. Many "new age" people and those in the modern wellness industry feel entitled to mimic and exploit Indigenous culture. We see mockeries of Indigenous ceremonies on reality TV or on social media every day. We see the corporate world selling "sage kits" as if sacred medicines are a lifeless commodity. Millions of people still see Indigenous spiritual culture as a plaything, a gimmick, or something that can simply be bought, sold, and disposed of. When Indigenous people ask for cultural appropriation to stop, we are often met with aggressive defensiveness. People say, "We respect you—it's a cultural exchange." But remember that "cultural exchange" wasn't an option for us for hundreds of years. The power structure remains imbalanced, so it can only be an exchange when it's on Indigenous terms.

We hope that if you are interested in learning from Indigenous spirituality, we have not dismissed you but rather have invited you in to understand the reality of how complex the task of cultural continuity and reclamation has been. We hope that you can now work with us as allies—something we greatly need during a time when the wellness industry is making billions of dollars from spiritual colonialism, all the while remaining oblivious and unhelpful when it comes to the economic hardships, health disparities, and other social ills that Indigenous communities continue to face because our ceremonies were outlawed for so long. We hope not only to educate people about the harms of spiritual theft and cultural appropriation, but also to offer an avenue for all people to practice true ally-ship, and to support Indigenous cultural revitalization in meaningful ways. There is power for all in understanding this truth.

Demonstrating Restraint as a Form of Respect

Instead of participating in any wellness activity that promotes and exacerbates appropriation, consider taking up the practice of truly honoring other cultures by showing restraint and abandoning feelings of entitlement. This doesn't mean that cultural exchanges have to stop; it simply means that they should be done with care, ensuring that everyone is respected. In our own lives and wellness journeys, we have learned so much and have grown spiritually by meeting people from other backgrounds. We can acknowledge that these relationships have enriched our lives, without having to go so far as to adapt or claim authority for all of these teachings.

For example, we have both taken many yoga courses over the years and learned a great deal about breathwork, asanas, and moving the mind with the body, but we do not claim expertise in or authority regarding this cultural practice from India that we were not raised with. This means that although we sometimes practice yoga or incorporate asanas into our movements, we do not consider ourselves to be yoga teachers or "yogis," and we respectfully remain silent during Sanskrit chants if the teacher has not taken the time to introduce the class to the meaning behind the words. Outside of practice, we have read articles to learn about the colonization of yoga, the differences between ancient yogic knowledge and the yoga industry in the West, and other ways that this practice has become widely misunderstood and taken out of context in recent decades.

Using restraint and understanding when to limit oneself spiritually are just as important as opening the heart and mind to accept new teachings. This is not to say that we are adamantly against the decision of any non-Indian person who has become a yoga teacher. Surely there are Indian institutions that have shared the practice widely, and we do not intend to undermine their authority on the matter. This is only to say that we are mindful of the decolonizing yoga conversation that is currently being led by the Indian community, and that we approach the practice with careful thought and consideration of how to practice it respectfully. Ultimately, just because we are spiritual people ourselves, we do not feel like we have to have access to or ownership of any and all spiritual knowledge. No one should feel so entitled.

Walking in a Ceremonial Way

All people are invited to *walk in a ceremonial way*, which is a profound method of incorporating daily ceremony into our lives and wellness practices. Similar to the benefits of elevating routine to ritual, this is a simple, nonperformative, and practical way to weave ceremony into the otherwise mundane aspects of life. When we walk in a ceremonial way,

- we avoid gossip, saying bad things about others, and engaging with or spreading rumors.
- we take time for silence, meditation, and walks outdoors.
- we make it a point to attend community gatherings, and we help out when we can.
- we avoid using foul language, especially in front of children (Indigenous languages did not include cursing).

- we are mindful of our words and their effects, especially paying attention to the first and last things we talk about at night, or what we talk about over food.
- we insert intention into everyday tasks, praying and expressing gratitude in our minds as we cook, clean, exercise, or wash our faces and brush our teeth.
- we do a "giving of thanks" with our kids before they fall asleep, talking with them about what and who they are grateful for.
- we teach our children how to greet plants, the sun, and the birds that fly by our windows.

These are small but mighty actions that, when done regularly, become the fabric of a steady, spiritual life. This is living each day like a ceremony.

A Resource for Allies

> Enormous amounts of time, energy, and money were spent eradicating our language and culture, and equal levels of resources and intentionality must be invested into language revitalization and cultural preservation.
>
> —*Rosebud Prosperity*

Many schools, organizations, and nonprofits are doing the hard work of reclaiming Indigenous spirituality, languages, and cultural teachings in Native communities today, teaching Indigenous children that they have the freedom to be proud of who they are and ensuring that they have access to critical healing tools that are still needed for them to live full and happy lives and to recover from historical trauma. We invite anyone to connect with, learn about, and donate to any Native-led Indigenous language immersion schools or nonprofit organizations in Indian Country that work tirelessly every day to ensure that Indigenous youth have opportunities to reconnect and remain rooted in their cultural teachings. Supporting these institutions of cultural revitalization is a true act of solidarity with Indigenous communities.

TAKE ACTION: HOW TO RESTORE BALANCE THROUGH CEREMONY

Learn

- What, if any, spiritual, religious, or ceremonial practices and rituals are a part of your familial and cultural heritage and history?
- Who can you respectfully ask to mentor, guide, or teach you more?
- Seek out books, classes, organizations, or other resources that can teach you more about a spiritual pursuit.
- Meditation can be a form of ceremony. Discover the many different modalities of meditation and research how you can learn these techniques from people who are certified to teach them.
- What occurrences, celestial events, and milestones that are important to you can you honor through ceremony? This can be a new ceremony created by you or one that has been revitalized from your ancestry.
- When adopting new spiritual practices that were not historically conducted by your family, ask yourself whether this ceremony or spiritual practice is appropriate for you to adopt.
- What medicines did your people use, and how can you begin to learn to respectfully access them?
- Part of bringing ceremony into your life entails respecting the spiritual practices of other groups of people. If you're living on the land of other Indigenous people, be sure to learn about which locations are sacred to them and how you can respect the spiritual and cultural privacy of those people. All land is sacred, so you can choose which areas on the land feel special to you.

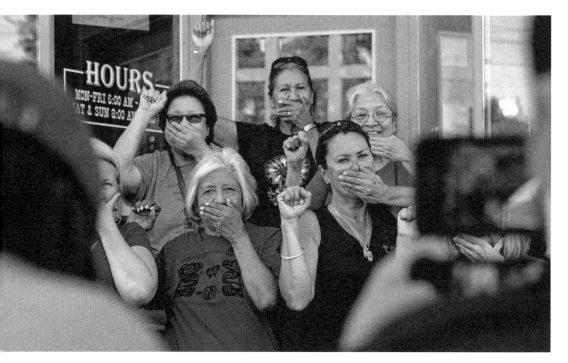

A group of Native women raise their fists and cover their mouths to represent advocacy for the ongoing epidemic of Missing and Murdered Indigenous Women, Girls, and Two Spirit people (MMIWG2S). Native people everywhere are reclaiming our power and voices after many generations of being shunned and silenced by the US and Canadian governments.

Engage

- Approach spirituality on a macro level—through worldview, perspective, and lifestyle. Approach it on a micro level as well—such as incorporating a few minutes of breathing exercises here and there.
- If you are learning about a spiritual practice that comes from outside of your culture, do everything you can to prioritize demonstrating respect and avoiding cultural appropriation. Tread lightly and be sure to hear a breadth of perspectives.
- After you have learned about creating or revitalizing ceremony, begin experimenting with applying it to your life to honor events that are important and sacred to you or to practice daily.

- Make it a priority to attend the ceremonies happening in your community.
- Assess how your overall wellness may or may not have improved. Ceremony should help bring us a sense of peacefulness and/or a sense of wholeness and productivity. If you feel good about the ceremonial practice you've applied to your wellness journey, then continue to use it and learn how it can evolve or become a new tradition in your family.
- Try different forms of meditation. Like anything, meditation takes time to learn, so you might not feel its positive effects right away. Be patient and keep meditating.
- Experiment with different times of the day or week or year to practice ceremony; find out what times work best for your lifestyle. For example, maybe meditation is best in the morning as soon as you wake up before having coffee, preparing for work, or getting the kids ready for their days. Maybe once a week you spend quality time sitting quietly in a ceremonial way to give thanks for things you're grateful for.
- Experiment with the practice of sitting in silence in a calm space; quiet the mind and visualize a positive version of yourself. How do you want to think, feel, and act in the future? Having a vision is an important piece in your journey of healing. Health and wellness are very much about continuing to grow and evolve into a healthier version of yourself—which then affects your family and community. Once you uncover your true self, set goals to begin to step into your truth.

Optimize

- You have been consistent with bringing ceremony into your life and have been able to notice the difference in your overall sense of well-being. Your outlook is more positive, and you're in the habit of being grateful.
- Your spiritual worldview has expanded, allowing you to observe the spiritual aspects of your life experiences.
- You have discovered which times are best for you to incorporate ceremonial practices into your life. Continue to practice them.

- The ceremony you've revitalized or created has become a tradition in your family, creating healthy relationships and improving an overall sense of well-being in all of its members.
- You've been attending ceremonies in your community or region and feel a sense of belonging and spiritual wholeness.
- Your spiritual wisdom has grown, and after some years, you may be asked to take on a role in facilitating ceremony in your community.
- You feel confident enough to teach family and friends how they can bring ceremony into their lives.
- You are contributing to an Indigenous organization that is committed to restoring spirituality for their youth.

INTERSECTION WITH OTHER CIRCLES

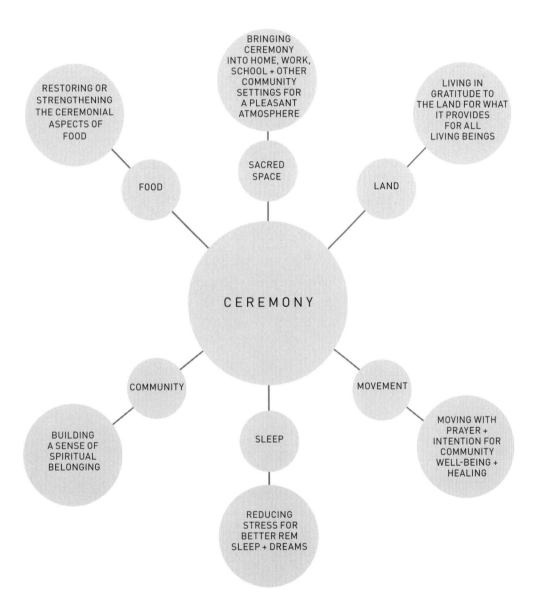

BRINGING CEREMONY INTO HOME, WORK, SCHOOL + OTHER COMMUNITY SETTINGS FOR A PLEASANT ATMOSPHERE

RESTORING OR STRENGTHENING THE CEREMONIAL ASPECTS OF FOOD

LIVING IN GRATITUDE TO THE LAND FOR WHAT IT PROVIDES FOR ALL LIVING BEINGS

FOOD

SACRED SPACE

LAND

CEREMONY

COMMUNITY

MOVEMENT

BUILDING A SENSE OF SPIRITUAL BELONGING

SLEEP

MOVING WITH PRAYER + INTENTION FOR COMMUNITY WELL-BEING + HEALING

REDUCING STRESS FOR BETTER REM SLEEP + DREAMS

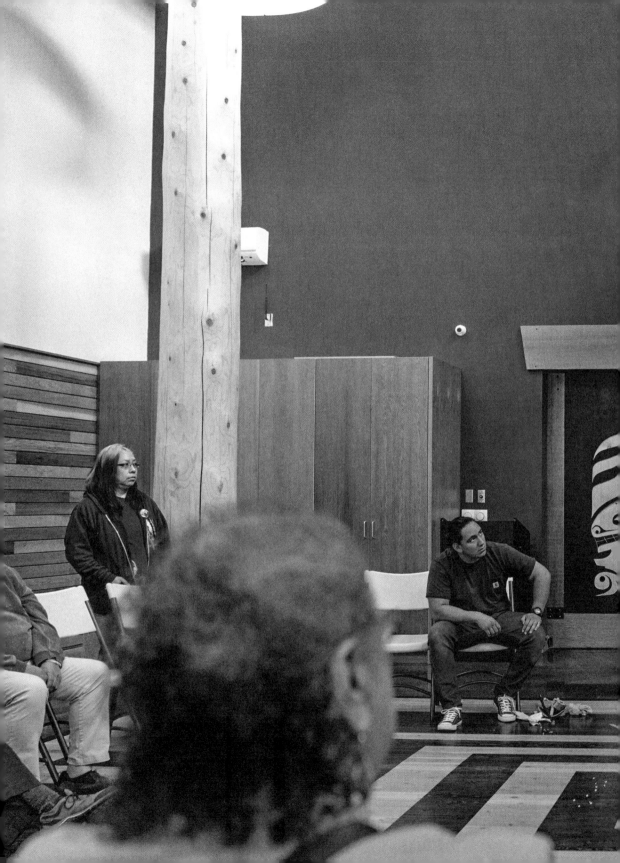

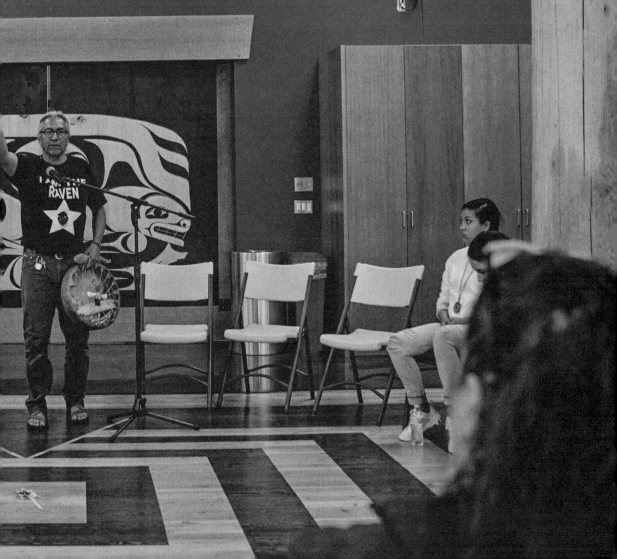

5

SACRED SPACE

Wherever you live, and whatever you live in, even if it is a one-room shack, or tent, or tipi, take care of it and try to make it look pretty and nice . . . You live there, and it represents your mother.

—*Celane Not Help Him, Lakota elder, in* Honor the Grandmothers: Dakota and Lakota Women Tell Their Stories

I choose the places where I live in a very scrupulous manner. There must be room for development and germination of the expectant forces that inevitably come to seek me out in my occupied rooms . . . I must dwell in places where I am always in awe of God and mortal men.

—*T. C. Cannon, Kiowa artist*

A PEACEFUL SPACE IS A PEACEFUL EXISTENCE

In this chapter, you will learn that the objects and environment that surround you as you cook in the kitchen or do stretches in the living room are not separate from the rest of your wellness journey but are an integral part of the practice that deeply impacts how you think, feel, and move. If you haven't thought yet about the opportunity to find healing through tending to your home, office, digital world, or other spaces where you spend time, this might just be the piece of the puzzle that will pull you in to a more balanced, relaxed state of being.

Previous spread: At the Skokomish Community Center, Gene Tagaban (Tlingit, Filipino, Cherokee) offers a prayer and song for healing and wellness as Josh Cocker (left) and Shalene Joseph (Aanih, Athabascan) (right) join in facilitating a wellness gathering for the Native Wellness Institute. This community space is carefully designed and cared for in a way that facilitates and supports the well-being of the nation.

CURATING SACRED HOMES

The Lakota lived in masterpiece tipis that followed the buffalo herds across the Great Plains, while the O'odham carved out cool desert homes from cactus rib and adobe clay. The Mandan and Hidatsa collaborated with the hills of their home country to build warm and inviting earth lodges, and the Haudenosaunee lived, worked, and prayed in grand timber longhouses. The Inuit made warm and inviting iglus of ice, while the Ojibwe built birchbark wigwam with balsam and cedar floors to purify and insulate the air. Indigenous people have always taken pride in keeping beautiful, functional, and sustainable homes. Our ancestors understood the ways that their living spaces and environment impacted their well-being.

Today, we must revitalize the teaching that a home is an extension of our well-being. We should once again begin to treat our homes as sacred spaces. Too often, we think of the places where we live, work, and hang out as objects or unliving buildings that do not affect our health. But the opposite is true. We sleep, cook, eat, raise babies, and spend countless hours under our own roofs, so we should have reverence for our homes and their rooms. When we put love and intention into creating safe and serene environments, those spaces can become family sanctuaries. A sacred home is thoughtfully designed and arranged in a way that facilitates all other aspects of our total well-being. This is how our ancestors viewed the spaces they occupied, and this is how we can view our homes, schools, and workplaces today. Expanding the concept of space, we can also consider our personal care processes and our digital spaces as extensions of our environment that influence our health, well-being, and sense of balance.

A home, or any other space, should be cared for not just in terms of physical maintenance, but in terms of spiritual maintenance. Often, when a Native family moves into a new home, or a person begins a new job in a new office, the first thing that we do is smudge (or ask an elder to come in and smudge) the space for us. At this time, we offer prayers for good, productive things to happen in the home. It is also common for Native families to keep sacred medicines on kitchen tables or nightstands so that anyone who comes into the home can smudge if they choose. We also encourage our children to smudge when they wake up in the morning or before they go to bed at night. This act of spiritual cleansing is a regular part of our culture that acknowledges the power of maintaining good thoughts and intentions for a physical dwelling. It is an understanding that these thoughts and intentions can turn into action, leading toward a state of living and working that is more productive, more emotionally in tune, and safer.

As we discussed in chapter 4, we do not encourage a universal use of smudging with Indigenous sacred medicines, as using medicine that one does not have a relationship with is considered cultural appropriation. However, we understand that there are ways of "making smoke" or cleansing a room that come from many cultures around the world—from burning incense, to lighting candles, to simply cleaning and opening a window with good and careful thoughts—and we encourage you to find a process that is true to you. All people can find a meaningful way to set a prayerful intention within their space and to acknowledge its sacredness.

Through stories, oral tradition, and historical accounts, we have learned about how our ancestors from many different nations kept their spaces sacred in precolonial times. Although no specific practice is ubiquitous across all tribes, there are some common themes. In order to keep a space that facilitates wellness, one can cleanse it, as discussed, or one can keep fresh air and sunlight circulating throughout it. To create a sacred space, it is also important to be mindful of the media that are playing and filling the airspace. It is important to avoid too much violence, noise, and otherwise disturbing or depressing content. One can incorporate the use of natural materials and plants as well. Finally, having clutter-free and minimal homes is an Indigenous virtue that many are turning to today.

It is not realistic to expect ourselves or anyone else to live exactly as our ancestors lived. The knowledge that they carried, the economies they maintained, the abundance of the landscapes that they preserved, and many other circumstances that were present then are simply not available today, so mimicking their existence is simply not feasible. What we can do, however, is adapt an ancestral mindset, taking into consideration the intentionality, the worldview, and the methods by which our ancestors kept their spaces sacred, and we can try to apply these to home, work, school, and any other indoor spaces. In this way, we can intentionally try to create spaces that facilitate wellness and balance.

In our home, we do not live in near-perfect symbiosis with the land and surrounding environment, as our ancestors did. Right now, we are renting a house in the suburbs where we have not met most of our neighbors; we rely on city recycling and sanitation programs; we are confined within four walls; and we would be very uncomfortable without running water and air-conditioning. We are creatures of capitalism, of contemporary American life, and of comfort. And yet, we have still found ways to create some semblance of a sacred space. We are doing our best within our contemporary circumstance, and we encourage others to do the same.

The steps we take to mimic our ancestors' reverence for home-space are quite simple. Since we are confined within four-walled rooms, we keep our windows wide open so that light and air can pour in to enliven and freshen up the space, which then invigorates our own life-breath and energy. We make an effort to bring the surrounding desert landscape into our home by creating dried plant arrangements, by stocking our cupboards with Indigenous foods that we have harvested from the land, by using baskets that are woven from native grasses, and by hanging landscape photographs on our walls. We inspire ourselves by keeping books and art that represent our heritage, our history, our passions, and the places and people we love. Instead of having a TV as the focal point of our living room, which would be too tempting to flick on and get lost in, we keep an array of comfortable chairs and floor pillows for visiting and moving so that we can stay present and active with one another. Instead of filling our garage with storage bins full of excess, we give away what does not fit in our closets, and we have turned our garage into a neatly organized gym—a worthy investment made during the coronavirus pandemic. Because sobriety is part of our wellness practice and spiritual beliefs, we do not allow alcohol in our home. Instead, we are stocked up on sparkling water, fresh fruits, coffees, and teas so that we can serve and enjoy delicious, nourishing drinks that do not make anyone sick. When we go to sleep at night, we leave all electronic devices outside the bedroom in order to facilitate good rest and to welcome the guidance that we may receive in the dream state. We also co-sleep with our daughters, because our ancestors always kept children close at night.

These are just some of the ways that we have consciously curated a sacred home that works for us and feels authentic and true to our culture and values, even in the absence of ideal circumstances. The way that you cultivate and arrange your own sacred home might be very similar or completely different from how we do things, and that is okay. We simply encourage an application of intention.

Sometimes we look out the window and feel a bit depressed by the vast exploitation that surrounds us. We are keenly aware of how recently, how abruptly, and how violently the land that we now live on, Akimel O'odham territory, was transformed into a sprawling, polluted city from the unending, biodiverse agricultural haven it used to be. Sometimes we drive by a rundown strip mall and can't help but joke around: "*This* is what they've done with the land?"

But inevitably we shake off the bitter feeling and try to focus on the positive. At least we can hear the birds chirping. At least we can see the sky above. At least we are culturally rooted, with an awareness, a commitment, and a goal to remake the world into a better place—and many good people all around us are doing the same. Despite all of the corruption and negativity in the world, we still have the agency to do our part in our own home. Remembering this gives us a small sense of control and comfort.

We are grateful for where we currently live, but like many people, we dream of a space that is even more special for our family. We currently own a one-acre plot of land on the Salt River Reservation, near the home where Thosh grew up, where we plan to build a forever-home that our daughters will eventually inherit. We are already envisioning the ways that we can break out of conventional American design to create a home that honors our heritage, our values, our taste, and the environment. We hope to incorporate desert materials like adobe and cactus rib; and ceremonial elements, like a meditation room and a door that faces east (an ancestral rule for O'odham homes). Ideally, we would include eco-friendly construction, such as having solar panels and paying careful attention to window size and ceiling height. We hope for it to be an indoor-outdoor space, one that feels seamlessly a part of the land that surrounds it. We have researched and found an Indigenous architect who has assisted us with blueprints. Her design takes into consideration our lifestyle of wellness, outdoor living, and our intertribal Indigenous heritage. We are envisioning a small but solid storytelling, sensory, and healing space that serves not just as the backdrop to our lives, but as a character in our intergenerational family story.

Our ability to dream of this home, and to know that it is a possibility in our future, is an immense privilege that we do not take for granted. We want to be clear that even without the prospect of building a home exactly as desired, any space can be revered, sacred, serene, and special. Indeed, there are those who live in a tiny corner of a bedroom who put their love, care, and intention into that area in a very powerful way; and there are also those who own a multitude of massive, expensive properties who place precisely zero spiritual love into the environment. It doesn't matter how much money you have, or how much stuff you own—your home can be a deep personal escape from the often chaotic outside world.

Just as we prioritize physical movement and eating well, prioritizing the creation of a sacred space will impact all other aspects of our wellness journey in a positive way. We often only subconsciously realize what our ancestors and Western science alike have shown: that everything about the way we arrange, organize, and style our homes affects our physical, mental, spiritual, and emotional well-being. Of each of the Seven Circles of Wellness, sacred space might be the one that can be most immediately addressed, leading to instant gratification, mental clarity, and emotional benefit. For example, it takes only a few minutes to make your bed each morning. And although you won't stand there staring at your made bed all day, you will know in the back of your mind that you have a comfortable, clean area to return to when you go to rest at night, and this can bring you peace of mind. Establishing a sacred space through minimalism, decluttering, cleansing, and mindfully decorating can help us to feel in control, can bring a sense of daily rejuvenation, and can free space in the mind to express emotions and to concentrate on other tasks. When we respect and revere our spaces, we respect and revere our own energy.

HOW SACRED SPACE HEALS
⊕   Sacred Space Medicine Wheel   ⊕

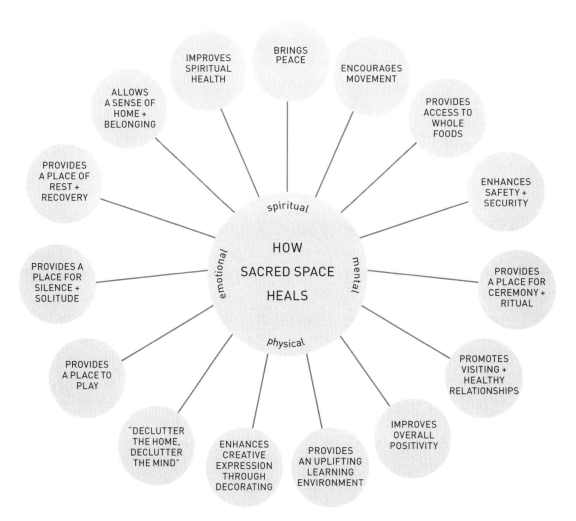

SPIRITUAL

Indigenous cultures typically do not separate places of prayer, spirituality, and reverence from places of living, working, and hanging out. Indeed, the sacredness of all spaces, indoor and outdoor, is understood. Today, we can practice minimalism, intentional design, and maintenance of our homes to facilitate peacefulness and serenity.

EMOTIONAL

Allowing natural light and fresh air to circulate indoors are two key components of ancestral Indigenous home design that are often absent from the artificially lit, boxed-in homes of today. When we open shades and windows, allowing the elements into our indoor spaces, our emotional health improves, thanks to the healing benefits of Mother Earth.

MENTAL

Our minds are often distracted by and preoccupied with the incessant visual and aural noise of televisions, computers, and other electronic devices. It is no wonder that most people feel the need to escape from home in order to clear their thoughts. By minimizing noise and valuing silence as our ancestors did, we can make our homes a place where deep thought, fulfilling conversation, and mindfulness can thrive once again.

PHYSICAL

Today, constantly exposed to advertisements, we are tempted to fill our lives and homes with stuff—often more than we need. We then neglect to leave open spaces in which we can move our bodies. Indigenous decluttering means leaving space for movement. When we know that we can move in our living space—not just in a gym away from our home—we facilitate a more consistent movement practice for ourselves, encouraging an active lifestyle for the whole family.

INDIGENOUS MINIMALISM: GENEROSITY IS WEALTH

There was no possible excuse for hoarding; on the contrary it stood for selfishness and lack of self-restraint, since all goods or accumulated property were tacitly for the purpose of distribution.

—*Luther Standing Bear,* Land of the Spotted Eagle

Today, people everywhere are turning to minimalism. They are buying less to prioritize long-term financial goals; they are shopping less to save time and energy; and they are accumulating less in the interest of the environment. These are wonderful efforts that we encourage. Our ancestors also practiced minimalism, but in a slightly different way. In precolonial times, across a diverse swath of tribal nations, one common theme permeated material culture and home life: generosity meant wealth. Those who owned the fewest things and gave the most away were the most respected. This concept made practical sense, especially for nomadic nations. The more items a family owned, the more they would have to carry when they moved camp. Too much stuff would be a burden. This is a far cry from the American culture of consumerism that encourages us to buy, buy, buy, leading to a false and very temporary sense of fulfillment and cluttered houses that bring daily stress.

In ancestral Indigenous homes, the line between art, generosity, and utility was often blurred. Museum curators continue to grapple with the question of "art" versus "artifact" when labeling Indigenous material culture, because indeed even the most mundane of items were exquisitely crafted. All items for daily use were finely decorated while also durable and made to last: spoons were carved of buffalo horn, tipi exteriors were painted to tell elaborate family histories, rugs and food-gathering baskets were woven by artistic masters. Every family prioritized safety, comfort, and cleanliness for all residents and visitors. Every home had a role in the larger community, and every person took pride in contributing to the home. This is a philosophy of living that we must return to today.

Part of creating a sacred space includes being welcome and generous. You might have a lot of beautiful decorations, but do you have some items on hand that are available to give as gifts when visitors come over? You might have a gorgeous kitchen with the latest appliances, but are you inviting people to eat with you? Ask yourself: Is my home a place where I am free to move my body, where my kids can dance and play, where singing and instruments are alive, where nourishing foods are being cooked, where I can find time for peace and quiet, and where I can find outdoor space to connect with the land, sky, and sun? Here, am I inspired by books and art that heal me and motivate me? These are some of the questions whose answers will help you to find what you need for creating a sacred space. We spend so much time in our homes that indeed they should feel like a sanctuary, not like a chaotic trap that we want to escape from.

NESTING FOR OUR NEWBORN
CHELSEY

Cheenugwun's wife cleaned the lodge, replacing the floor covering with cedar boughs and re-arranging the household bundles. Their godson must breathe in the sweet scent of cedar and look upon order and cleanliness. Perhaps the child would somehow absorb a sense of beauty and harmony.

—An Ojibwe family's ritual before meeting a newborn relative,
from Ojibwe Ceremonies

When we found out we were pregnant with our firstborn, Alo, we were living in a very tiny condo in Old Town, Scottsdale, Arizona. As our pregnancy went on, we became determined to transform our space from the haphazard layover pad of traveling freelancers to a comfortable home fit for a baby. I

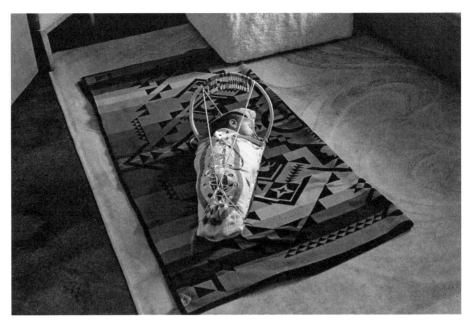

Westyn (seven months old) takes an afternoon nap in her cradleboard at home. The cradleboard, a baby carrier used by many different tribes, facilitates comfort and healthy growth for the baby. Hers was originally made for her older sister, Alo, in a collaborative effort by her grandparents and great-aunt. It will stay in the family for generations.

was stunned to find that the "nesting" instinct you hear about is not only real, but quite powerful. My quest to cozy up the apartment started out as an urge, and then became a mission.

Triggered by hormones, I discovered that there is something deeply engrained in our humanity that calls us to keep our dwellings safe, clean, and beautiful in a way that pleases our senses and protects our families. My hypothesis is that because I was very in tune with my body, mind, and emotions in other ways—focusing on proper nutrition, movement, and peacefulness—I was able to feel this nesting instinct to its fullest. Intentional home-keeping, I thought, is a sacred expression of love, and I was bound to follow through for my baby.

I was so excited when I found out I would be a mom, but maybe more than that, I was afraid. Suddenly I was faced with all of my inadequacies, and I didn't know whether I was prepared for the ultimate responsibility of bringing a precious little life into the world. As the pregnancy progressed, and I had more time to think about every possible complication or outcome, my fears continued to grow. Since I am a person who struggles with anxiety anyway, the idea of raising a child could seem like too big a responsibility to bear. But the process of nesting and preparing my space gave me an instant sense of grounding and control. It became an invaluable aspect of taking care of my mental health while pregnant.

I started by decluttering. I emptied our closets and cabinets, donated what was usable and threw out what was not usable, and then refolded and reorganized everything that remained. When that was done, I moved on to decorating. I didn't have a big budget, but I found a few landscape photos taken by Thosh, as well as a few poems and art prints I had collected over the years, and I placed them in vintage frames to hang above our bed. I brought in houseplants to bring life into the home and to cleanse the air. I took out chemical-smelling cleaners and soaps and replaced them with unscented, nontoxic options.

We had only two bedrooms in the condo, and one was being used for our office, so instead of having a separate nursery (which wouldn't have felt right anyway—the Indigenous tradition is to co-sleep), we made a little corner for our baby in our room with her own dresser, changing table, and special decorations. Because space was limited, I put especially careful thought into choosing what would go on her wall. Blending form with function, I chose two rustic metal wall hooks with blue stone detail on which to hang her swaddle blankets and wrap carrier. I fastened them to the wall just so, and felt so much satisfaction each time I grabbed a clean blanket from those hooks. Above the other side of the changing table, we placed sweetgrass and sage so that our medicines to smudge as a family would be easily accessible.

In the end, nothing was fancy, but everything felt intentional and purposeful. I looked around with pride: I had created a sacred space that was fit for our sacred little baby.

Today in our home, we have a bit more space, but we still try not to fill our home with stuff. Our commitment to clutter-free living remains. We own only as much as we need, plus some extras here and there of things that contribute to our health. A creative, well-thought-out space helps us feel peaceful and clearheaded. When our home makes sense and feels safe, the world around us feels safer, too.

LET IN THE SUNLIGHT
THOSH

When I was growing up, I often heard adults talking about the work of medicine people around the O'odham communities. Just as with Western medicine and doctors, there are also specialists among Native healers. Some specialize in diagnosing the root of "spiritual trauma," others heal the physiology of the body, and still others specialize in medicinal plants and herbs or medicines that come from the animal nations. When I was young, one medicine woman was particularly well-respected. She was often called upon by various O'odham families, or to help with community gatherings; she was always generous with her time and energy, responding to the needs of others. Out of respect for her family's privacy, I will call her Mrs. H.

Several times, I heard Mrs. H talk about her work of doctoring people. When she spoke about this, everyone listened intently, because she had a very specific gift of sensing unseen forces that would prey upon people and make them sick. There was always something to learn from her about spiritual health. She did not do her work in front of too many people, but those who witnessed it were sometimes amazed, and always satisfied with the results. Mrs. H would tell us that when she visited people's homes, she would doctor not only the person, but sometimes the whole family and the house.

She is the person who taught me that our well-being is directly influenced by the health of the spaces we find ourselves in. I have since learned that this is a shared belief in many other parts of the Indigenous world. Native healers have long recognized that not only does the patient carry the burden of disease and suffering, but so does the family, even if they don't realize it. (The same goes for the opposite, of course. When a person is well, it is reflected in their family and home.)

Mrs. H instructed her patients to open the windows and let in the sunlight. She spoke about the importance of sun to our spiritual and emotional health. The sunlight is sacred, a helper, and a life-giver. Inviting it into our homes is integral to maintaining healthy spaces. She also brought attention to the TV and advised against watching violence, gore, or horror. She was especially adamant about this in regards to young children, because their minds can be negatively impacted by such content. Some studies are now showing that disturbing content can arouse emotions of fear, anxiety, and shock that negatively affect the psychological health of children.[1] This is one of many areas of medicine that Indigenous healers were already well aware of before Western science began to take notice.

Mrs. H and her helpers utilized very specific procedures for asking bad forces to leave the home to allow healing for the family. She always reminded us that her work "wasn't magic"; the family played a role in the healing and had a responsibility to continue to do her work and follow up with everyday maintenance. It's just like Western medicine—when a patient is sick, a doctor can prescribe medication or perform surgery, but it's up to the patient to make lifestyle changes for health. Indigenous medicine, too, is interwoven with our daily actions and habits.

Many Indigenous families sought spiritual help because of inherited and unresolved grief, which sometimes led to a pattern of addiction or domestic violence. It is commonly understood among various Indigenous nations that when people exhibit these behaviors, negative energy comes into the home, exacerbating preexisting illness. Therefore, the family always needs to take into account the state of their home when making plans for undertaking a healing journey.

As I got older I was able to assist a group of people in my community who did home treatments, and I saw firsthand how the energy and cleanliness of a home could either contribute to a healthy life or further exacerbate preexisting illness or suffering. These experiences over the years influenced my understanding of the importance of maintaining good ways of housekeeping. When I was a bachelor in my twenties on my own healing journey, I knew that living in a minimal, organized, alcohol-free home went hand in hand with exercising my body, staying sober, working hard, creating art, treating others well, and all other aspects of a healthy life. Later, when we started our family, these teachings sank in even more, and I have realized just how critical a safe, clean home is for the healthy development and happy lives of children.

Every evening, I go through our house, close the blinds, and set an intention to keep my family safe and protected indoors after the sun goes down. We keep lighting very dim to prepare us for sleep time. In the morning, I am usually the first to wake up. Around 5:30 a.m. I go around the house and open the windows again, except for in our bedroom, because Alo, our oldest, likes that to be her first job of the day. When she wakes up, right away she says, "Open the light! Open the light!" We go to the blinds and open them together. "Hello, sun!" she says in her precious little voice, and together we begin the day. I feel very satisfied when I watch the girls play and toddle around our home in such a carefree manner. Chelsey and I feel accomplished in our parenting knowing we have created a space where our daughters feel safe, loved, carefree, and confident.

As a father and husband, I had to consciously reimplement many teachings that I had heard growing up, such as always knowing where my sacred items and medicines are, because you never know when you'll need to take them out to pray. This has helped our home stay spiritually well. Grounding ourselves, smudging, and praying are regular practices in our space, and we do them with intention. I also make sure to sing songs, another way to nurture good energy, using my hand drum and gourd as my instruments. I often sing traditional songs, but I have also created some new ones that came to me as I rocked each of the girls to sleep when they were newborns. I believe these songs were gifts to our family. So to honor these gifts, we continue to sing them to invite in positive feelings of family, renewal, and gratitude.

All activities like acoustic sound, song, dance, play, laughter, prayer, ceremony, smudge, silence, and cooking healthy food keep a continuous, positive energy circulating through our home that has a calming and loving effect on all who come to visit. Even as we were writing this book at home, before each writing session, we lit our smudges and gave thanks for a clear mind and good heart and prepared ourselves to be a hollow bone for good things to be written for you to read. When we needed breaks, we took moments to tidy up or rearrange our surroundings, opening space so that our minds and hearts could be open to work. We hope that these words and this advice bring you the clarity and comfort it has brought to us.

Trauma-Informed Decluttering

Just as Mrs. H recognized that darkness and negative activity in a home were the result of trauma, not the fault of an individual, we recognize that the conversation about sacred space should also be trauma-informed and free of judgment. Clutter, hoarding, or a home in disarray is often a reflection of very challenging circumstances that people have been through or are going through. Living in an unsafe home environment, being a trauma survivor, or living through high-stress experiences are all barriers to the amount of control that one has over one's space. Staying tidy requires energy and support, and not everyone has the same amount of those in their lives.

Sometimes, having a big, boisterous family is also a good reason for a home not being perfectly clean. This is not a bad thing! We understand it, because this is how we were raised—with lots of siblings in not-so-big homes. While there are many upsides to living with big families, there are also some challenges—one being that it is hard to find personal space and privacy. A large family makes it more difficult to keep common areas clean.

Large families are common in Indigenous communities and in many others. We encourage everyone to recognize the generosity that is required for taking in relatives, staying connected to extended family, and embracing those who need help or a place to stay. Even though it makes home-keeping more difficult, this is a part of modern life that is something to be proud of, not ashamed of.

While encouraging intentional decluttering, we remain aware that the opposite end of the clutter spectrum—an environment that is too rigid or uncomfortable—might be more harmful than helpful and can also be a trauma response. Just as with food or exercise, creating a clean, serene space is all about balance.

We know that our ancestors encouraged careful attention to a clean, well-kept space, and now science has also shown that a cluttered home can be a source of stress.[2] So it may help to begin viewing the idea of intentional home-keeping as an opportunity, not a chore. If you are feeling out of balance, this might be an area of your health that you have not yet thought to address. Feel free to abandon any sense of self-judgment and try your best to implement a solution. You can start small—

clean off a side table, tackle some laundry, or make your bed. Observe how good that feels, and continue to incorporate decluttering into your wellness routine. The goal is not to have a perfect home, but rather to know that a bit of home-keeping can lift your spirits, clear your mind, or give you a special kind of boost in your day.

PROTECT YOUR SPACE: BOUNDARIES AND SAFETY

Keeping boundaries in your space is a part of protecting yourself. This might look like not allowing negative people, things, or substances to enter. A participant in one of our workshops shared a profound story with us. For years, she had struggled to set boundaries with family members. She was often the person who would allow a down-and-out relative to crash on her couch for days or even months at a time. This habit of taking people in continued to bring chaos and drama to her and her family, and contributed to her own struggle with addiction and substance abuse. Finally, one day she got to a stage in her life when she had children and became very serious about sobriety. When she expressed to her social worker that she felt guilty about not allowing relatives to live with her anymore, he offered her some advice that stuck with her: "When you say no to someone toxic, you are saying yes to others who need you more—like your children."

In Indigenous culture, we particularly struggle with saying no to relatives sometimes, because generosity and keeping an open door have been central to our value systems for centuries. Today's world is a little more complicated, though, so this is an area where our ancestral values can't be simply cut and pasted. If you are in a position to take someone in without it interfering with the well-being of other vulnerable people in your home, or without it interfering with your own health, then that might be a noble and generous thing to do. But if the person in question cannot be trusted, or if you do not have the energy, the means, or the ability to set healthy boundaries, then remember that it is best to say no.

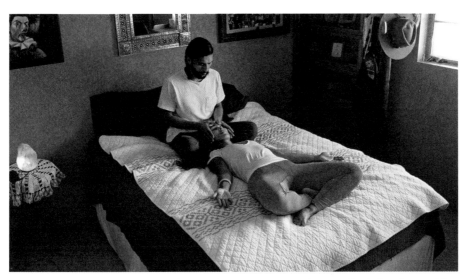

Quetzal Guerrero (a musician) and Sunshine Zerda (a yoga instructor), longtime family friends, exemplify healthy, holistic living. They take time to relax in their clean, well-lit, creative space.

Digital Smudge: Cleansing Your Virtual Space

In the 1970s, an Indigenous grandmother from Brazil, Clara Shinobu Iura, received a message from spiritual beings who alerted her to a destructive problem on the horizon. "They warned us that it is necessary to be attentive to products created by technology that can pollute and destroy our terrestrial atmosphere," she said. They told her that people are at risk of losing themselves in material and technological life.[3]

Today, seven in ten Americans are active on social media,[4] and there are nearly four billion internet users worldwide. Indigenous people are highly active in the digital world, just like anyone else. In fact, it seems that many marginalized groups have been especially active online, using social media as tools to take control of our own narratives and to engage in a new form of activism. Our ancestors may never have imagined what this digital world would look like, but similarly to other traditional teachings, their lessons on social codes, community values, and personal conduct remain relevant in this space. The digital world is a trickster. It can be useful, but it can also be a dreadful place that harms mental and emotional health—especially that of young people. Some have called it a public health crisis.[5] Today, if we are online, we must learn to metaphorically "smudge" or cleanse

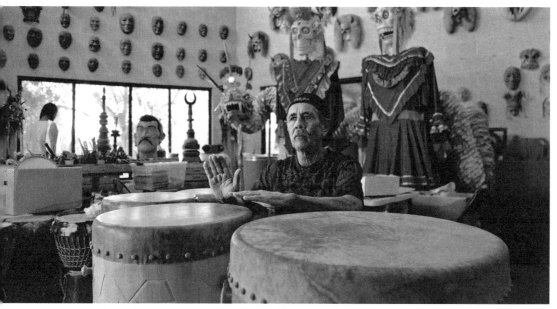

Zarco Guerrero, a mentor of Thosh's, plays his own hand-carved drums in his well-lit studio. It is important to him to have a space that facilitates his music and art, which he considers to be not only his work, but also his mode of ceremony and healing.

our digital space and to become more conscious and in control of the way that our online interactions impact our overall well-being.

Internet addiction is a real and growing problem. People are using technology to escape their day-to-day lives. For some, it has become a debilitating crutch that governs every aspect of their day.[6] With tech companies now pushing consumers toward virtual reality and the idea of life in the metaverse, it is predicted that rates of engagement and addiction will only grow, with great destructive potential for public health.[7] The best solution right now is prevention. Those of us concerned with maintaining balanced lifestyles can lead the conversation toward rooting oneself in the real world as a wellness practice. It starts with taking control of our own online behavior. This means getting serious about personal limits on screen time, being highly selective with how many social media platforms we engage with, refraining from joining every new digital trend, and, in general, taking plenty of time each day to simply be present in the real world.

Just as we do with our homes, we should be regularly decluttering our digital spaces, even in small ways. Our digital worlds are spaces to be monitored, cared for, and cleansed. We should be regularly decluttering our desktops—both the one the computer sits on and the one on the computer's screen. We should be mindful of how many tabs are open in our browsers. We should filter junk mail, unsubscribe from marketing emails, and regularly clear out our inboxes. Just as we have fitness routines and sleep schedules that we follow for our health, we can think of our digital structure as a system or policy that we take seriously for our health. If we establish a sense of control now, as individuals and as a society, we are more likely to face fewer health consequences in the future. Thankfully, we will always be able to glean advice from the value systems of our ancestors, whose teachings remain relevant in all spaces.

In general, ask yourself: Who will you allow into your virtual space? What type of energy are you exuding and absorbing? The mood, volume, and intensity of online interactions can impact overall wellness just as much as, if not more than, the real world does, and it is something that everyone can honestly evaluate and address accordingly. Remember to keep your digital space cleansed.

TAKE ACTION:
HOW TO CREATE A SACRED SPACE

Learn
- Learn about minimalism by watching documentaries or reading articles on the practice. Listen to stories about how minimalism has changed other people's lives.
- Learn about preindustrial architecture and other diverse forms of home design. Find a style that speaks to you.
- Learn about the benefits of natural sunlight, fresh air, and indoor plants.
- Read up on potentially harmful ingredients in personal care and cleaning products, and make careful decisions about what products feel right to use in your home and on yourself.
- Regarding digital spaces: think about the big picture of your life, and identify how much time and energy you want to be spending online.

Engage

- Identify an area in your home that you are willing to declutter. After doing one area, sit with the feeling of peace that it brings you, and then continue into the rest of your spaces.
- Thoughtfully set boundaries in your home, school, or workplace regarding safety, energy, and what types of activities take place there.
- If the process of giving away and decluttering items feels emotionally challenging, know that this is a perfectly normal response. Go at your own pace, take your time, and seek support from a friend or family member during this process.
- Center wellness in your home design and planning.
- Listen to music, watch movies, and read books that inspire and uplift you. Recognize the ways that the media you consume affect behavior, attitudes, and feelings of peace.
- Set an intention before day-to-day tasks like dusting, cleaning off your kitchen table, or making your bed, viewing these as opportunities to cleanse your headspace as well as your physical space.
- Care for plants, flowers, and herbs that you grow inside and outside of your home.
- Clean up and take care of outdoor areas and create space outside to sit, eat, hang out, or move.
- Remove phones and electronics from the bedroom so they do not interfere with sleep.
- Regarding digital space: work backward from the digital life picture that you have identified and begin drawing boundaries, setting time limits, and developing a system of control over your digital presence. Think of this as being as much a part of your health journey as exercise and eating well.

Optimize

- Your space feels serene, peaceful, and safe, and people comment on the good feelings they experience when they visit you there.
- You have created numerous spaces and nooks where you are free to move, which helps you seamlessly integrate a movement practice in any area of your home.
- Your home, school, or workplace is decluttered, clean, and welcoming.

- You regularly smudge or cleanse the air space in your home with fresh air, sunlight, and/or sacred medicines, whichever suits your lifestyle.
- You respect your space and it feels sacred to you, you have reverence for it, you care for it, and you love it.
- You are comfortable with your relationship to the digital world, and your time spent there is productive, not harmful or all-consuming.

INTERSECTION WITH OTHER CIRCLES

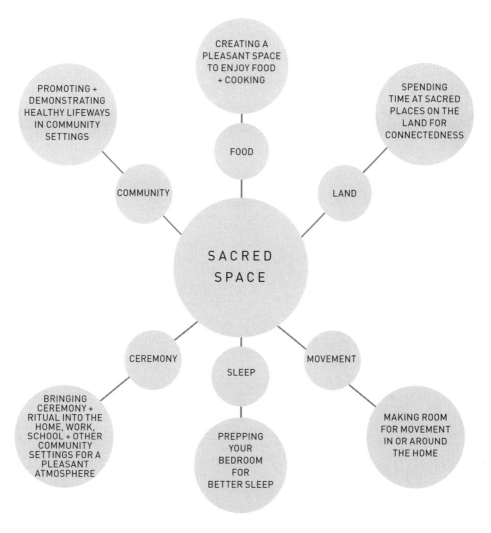

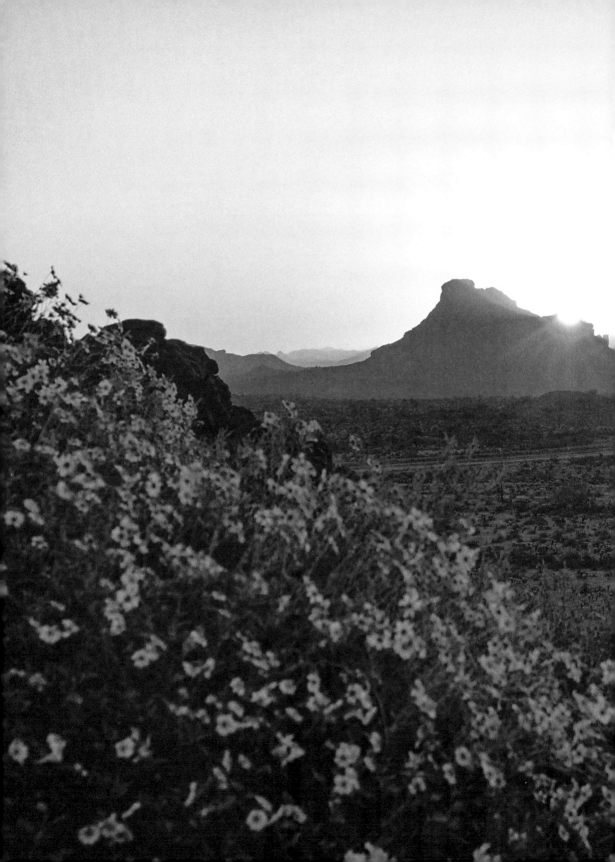

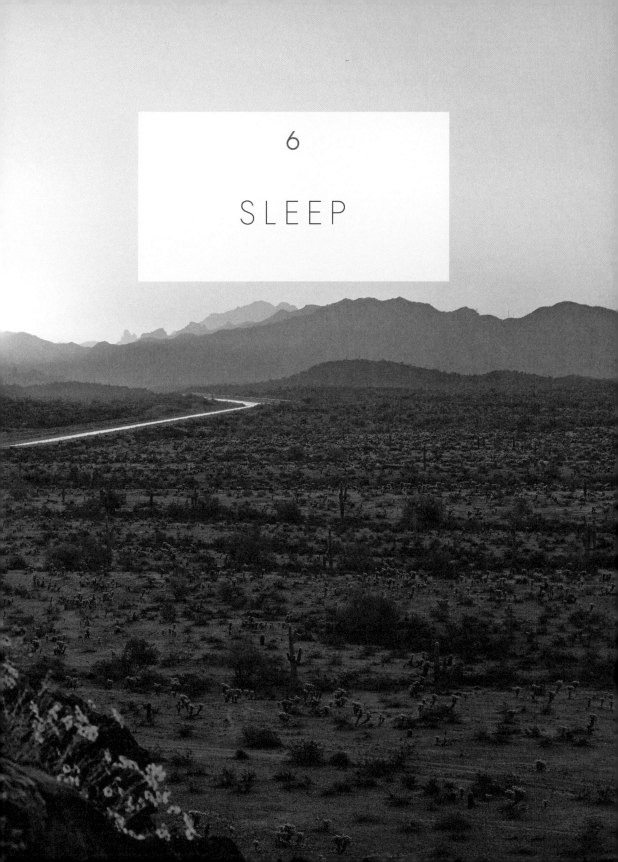

6

SLEEP

Once I heard an elder say, this is why we are having a hard time [achieving] the things we want. Our grandmother can no longer hear us or see us where we are sleeping. She cannot connect with us to share or give us a dream.

—*Ogimaagwaneebiik (Nancy Jones), Anishinaabe elder, on the shift from sleeping on the ground to sleeping on beds, from* Dibaajimowinan: Anishinaabe Stories of Culture and Respect

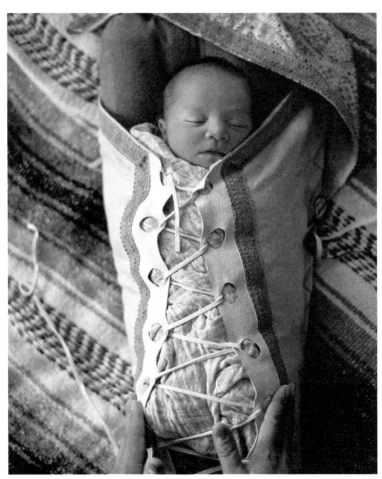

Alo (five days old) sleeps in her cradleboard. Following tradition, her auntie Naomi Clifford (Lakota, Osage, Seneca-Cayuga) was the first person to wrap her in it when she returned from the hospital.

A VISUALIZATION:
NIGHT AND DAY, PAST AND PRESENT

Envision a morning at home a few hundred years ago. It is springtime, the season of renewal and growth, and dawn is about to break. You sleep close to the earth, under the heavy comfort of buffalo robes, which offer a deep, protected rest. It's as if the mighty animal itself is guarding you through the night. With peace in body and mind, you regularly, fully enter deep sleep and a vibrant dream state. Because you do not use an overly cushioned mattress, the tiny muscles in your body have been massaged by the ground all night, and you wake up feeling limber and light. Your circadian rhythm is aligned with the rhythm of the earth because you have been gently conditioned since childhood to sleep with the stars and rise with the sun.

You are easily awoken in the morning by your keen senses feeling the shifting temperature outside. A new day does not alarm you, it excites you. You open your eyes and watch the smoke from the smoldering fire perform its effortless, acrobatic dance toward the opening at the top of the lodge. Your eyes move to a sharp ray of light seeping in, landing directly on the vessel of water hanging above your head. You sit up and take a sip. Clean, cold water. Your quickly scan your cozy home to see everything and everyone neatly and safely in their places. You are ready to get up. You put on your moccasins, crawl toward the door, and then take one last glance around the lodge before leaving. You notice the other members of your family are now beginning to stir. They will get up soon, too. With a smile of gratitude for the safety and presence of all, you softly step onto the fresh, dewy grass.

In the distance you hear the sound of the flowing river. The land that surrounds you is part of your home, not separate from it. You care for it and love it just as you love your lodge. You face the east to greet the sun, which by now has colored the sky a rosy pink, like the chubby cheeks of your newborn baby. You stand with good posture, presenting yourself respectfully to your surroundings.

Previous spread: The sun peeks over Red Mountain as dawn breaks—a sacred time for O'odham people.

Then you take a few deep, cold breaths, in through the nose, out through the mouth. Each inhale fills your body and works to energize the pump of your heart. This is all the stimulant you need, and before long, you are wide awake. You notice how the cool wind on your face conflicts with the growing warmth of the sun's rays. Everything is balanced.

As the rest of your relatives and neighbors begin to rise and emerge, few words are spoken. You politely allow everyone to begin the day with peaceful thoughts and silent prayers. Walking through your village, you use your smiling eyes to greet elders, children, friends, relatives, animals, plants, rocks, and fires. It is wonderful to bear witness to the beauty in your world. You are among a people who are proud to live in partnership with the land. What new stories will arrive in our nation today? You walk toward the water, listening more to the sounds of your people and your homelands. When you reach the river's edge, you put down some tobacco and offer thanks to Creator for this life, this land, and this day. You will make the most of it.

This was a morning in the life of our ancestors, who lived in a way that honored sleep and rest. As you move through this visualization, focus on all of the elements that work in concert to set the stage for good sleep. With good rest, the emotions and body are moved toward the beginning of a good day. Now, let's step into another peaceful iteration of life with ancestral sleep habits. This time it is summer, it is evening, and we are in the present day.

In the summertime in your home, you keep your windows wide open day and night, using natural light and air more often than their artificial counterparts, allowing your circadian rhythm to align with the outdoors. It is evening, and you check your phone for the last time after dinner, taking care to put away all blue-light devices a few hours before bed to prepare your mind for sleep. You are full, but not too full, from a hearty, simple meal of steak and wild rice with veggies. You won't wake up hungry in the middle of the night, nor will your fullness interfere with your rest. Earlier this morning, you did a short but effective kettlebell workout in your backyard. Because of this, your metabolism has continued to work all day, so by day's end, you are sufficiently tired.

You are sitting on the floor playing blocks with your kids as you watch the indoor light change with the sunset. You watch the dust dance in a beam of light that flashes across above the head of your toddler. You marvel at her cuteness, forgetting all about the tantrum she threw earlier. Instead of noise from the television in the background, you are playing your favorite instrumental music. Minutes later, the room is darker still, and you point out the window, asking your child what she sees. "It's the moon!" Yes, it's the moon, which means that we get ready for bed.

Your nighttime routine is always the same, bringing a comforting familiarity and making life easier on everyone. It is one less decision to make, one less complication. First we change into jammies, then we brush teeth, then we give thanks and smudge. Sometimes, the kids like to smudge their stuffed animals, especially Raccoon. Next, we crawl into bed for a book, or to recite a traditional story from memory. After the kids have adventures with *Where the Wild Things Are* or trained like warriors on their brave blue horse, dad sings a song while the babies fall asleep. They're off for more adventures in the dream world.

After one last peek at the faces of your precious little ones, you think about how grateful you are for their health and safety, and you begin your own nighttime routine. First, a quick cleanup around the house, which brings a sense of mental clarity. You dread the dishes, yet you do them because you have proved to yourself time and again that you feel better in the morning when you do not see them piled up in the kitchen. After tidying, you lock all the doors, shut off the ceiling lights, and turn on a few lamps instead. You go into the bathroom to brush your teeth and wash your face. As you splash water on your skin, you integrate a mental cleansing ritual, reminding yourself to let go of any bad feelings that came up over the course of the day. Skincare is another ritual. You consciously enjoy the smell, touch, and even temperature of the lotions or serums that you apply with care. As you pat them into your face, you remind yourself that you deserve this time.

After crawling into your crisp, clean sheets, you read for a few minutes and then talk to your partner—about anything. Days can be so busy. It is always a good thing to reconnect before sleep, expressing appreciation and care for one another. Before closing your eyes, you light the smudge on your bedside table and silently thank Creator for it all. Because you are sleeping so solidly, you begin to dream, receiving teachings and guidance from unknown entities. When you recall these dreams later, you do not expect a clear and logical interpretation; rather, you understand that these dreams are messages that guide you toward further questions in life. It is always good to embrace mystery, to pose questions to yourself, and to move through life with an openness to the wisdom that this mindset can bring. As you sleep, your muscles recover, your memory synthesizes, and you allow the brilliance of your body to take over. Sleep truly is a powerful form of healing.

HOW SLEEP HEALS
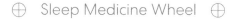
Sleep Medicine Wheel

SPIRITUAL

Sleep is a sacred time in which a person can tune in to receive guidance from their ancestors, Creator, and other unknown entities. With consistent good rest, a person can receive spiritual knowledge while in the dream world.

EMOTIONAL

The sun has always been honored by Indigenous peoples from all nations as a sacred and life-giving force that brings us joy, happiness, and renewal each day. When we are in tune with the rising and setting of the sun, we maximize vitamin D intake, thus feeling the sun's emotional healing benefit.

MENTAL

Waking up to greet the sun is the first step in sharpening the mind and preparing one's thoughts for a day of learning, creating, working, and listening. We must get out of the habit of waking up with our smartphones and replace it with the habit of stepping into or looking at the sun before we engage with artificial blue light.

PHYSICAL

Living in balance requires an understanding of oppositional energies and embracing each side. As we honor the sun and day, so we honor the night, stars, and moon. As we honor hard work, strenuous movement, and intellectual rigor, so we must also honor and prioritize rest. When we rest, our body has an opportunity to recover, and our muscles have an opportunity to grow.

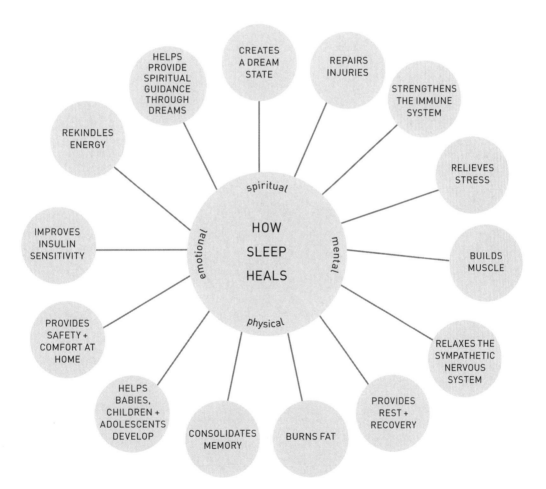

NT O S-GEVK MANT O S'AP KOI: "I'LL BE STRONG (TOMORROW) IF I GET A GOOD SLEEP" (O'ODHAM SAYING)

Sleep has been valued across all cultures throughout history, yet there are some distinctive features about how Indigenous people of the Americas thought about sleep. Oral tradition across Native Country teaches us that both sleep and the nighttime were greatly respected by our ancestors, revered as a spiritual time for rest and recovery. Our people were in tune with the sun and moon cycles, and their schedules deliberately followed them. As the sun went down, the people went in their homes and began to wind down for the night. People would lie down, begin to quiet their minds, and give thanks for what the day had brought to them. The dream world awaited them where sometimes they would be visited by relatives who had passed on to the spirit world.

For the most part, ancestral teachings emphasize the importance of staying indoors when it was dark, except during storytelling time, socials, or certain ceremonies. During those times people were advised to be near the fire. Fire is seen as a protector who keeps the people warm and safe. Many tribes have trickster stories that teach why we stay out of the dark. People knew that it was dangerous in the dark, and they also understood how important it was to be in a state of recovery, especially after a hard day's work. They knew that the next day would be filled with more tasks that their survival depended on, and so they needed to recoup physically and mentally. Today, telling someone that they need to stay in at night sounds superstitious, but it remains true that dangerous situations and getting into trouble still tend to happen at night.

In recent decades, neuroscience has uncovered the various mechanisms associated with different stages of sleep, helping us to understand how and why our bodies urge us to get good rest. Two internal biological mechanisms work together to regulate all functions of the body: circadian rhythms and homeostasis. Circadian rhythms synchronize with environmental cues to help control body temperature, metabolism, and the release of hormones. Meanwhile, sleep-wake homeostasis is our body's way of keeping track of the need for sleep. Factors that can disrupt our body's natural ability to fall asleep when we need sleep include working a night shift, exposure to light, medications, and stress.[1] In short, our bodies are brilliant at telling us when we need to sleep and even helping us to fall asleep, but our own resistance and lifestyle factors can prevent us from getting enough.

Newer research has revealed even more about the role of sleep for cognitive function. Memory consolidation happens during sleep, which is important for our learning, no matter how old we are. Most studies suggest that learning and memory depend on the quality and quantity of sleep.[2] In regards to Indigenous cultural and language preservation, and the passing on of the oral tradition, memory is everything, as much of our social and ceremonial gatherings require countless songs and dances and elaborate protocol to be enacted. Some creation stories are so long that they take days to recite. In order for stories, songs, dances, and languages to be passed on, we must maintain healthy cognitive functioning into our elderly years. Therefore, anyone who is interested in Indigenous cultural revitalization, or anyone who is interested in any type of academic pursuit or mentally rigorous career, must begin to view healthy sleep as a critical aspect to whole-life wellness.

Sleep affects our physical health as well. Our elders are always reminding us to get a good rest before a physically rigorous community function, like a ceremony or a social dance. Science tells us that during REM (rapid eye movement) sleep, we experience a number of different functions associated with muscle growth and recovery. Sleep is essential for weight management, as the most calories are burned during the REM stage, helping to reduce the incidence of diseases where obesity is a risk factor.[3] With a better quality of sleep, our immune systems become better at fighting infections because of the proteins, called cytokines, produced as we sleep.

Lack of Sleep

It is estimated that fifty to seventy million Americans suffer from chronic sleep disorders and wakefulness that hinder daily functioning, resulting in adverse health effects.[4] Some studies suggest that people all over the world are sleeping less than previous generations. The National Sleep Foundation suggests that most adults need seven to nine hours of sleep each night, yet data analyzed by the Centers for Disease Control and Prevention have shown that nearly 40 percent of adults are regularly getting fewer than seven hours each night.[5]

Today, every type of sleep-assisting technology is available, from countless mattress options to white noise machines. Yet it is because of other forms of technology, like personal electronic devices, streaming services, and social media platforms, that people are being exposed to increasing amounts of blue light before bedtime, which interferes with their sleep. A growing body of evidence suggests that blue light may suppress the body's production of melatonin, the hormone that prepares the body for sleep, keeping us in a wakeful state.[6] These new breakthroughs in sleep science are congruent with the concerns that traditional Indigenous medicine people have had, who often advise limiting electronic device usage and suggest being mindful of the content we are exposed to through them.

Corporate America promotes a culture of workaholics who are often expected to function on little to no rest. Often, people even boast about how little sleep they get and still carry on with their day. But research shows that poor-quality sleep, especially over the long term, leads to sleep disorders and a wide range of other negative health outcomes, including an increased risk of hypertension, diabetes, obesity, depression, heart attack, and stroke.[7] For instance, with regards to type II diabetes, poor sleep is associated with increased glucose levels, or blood sugar intolerance (which is a precursor to diabetes), and insulin resistance.[8] Sleep deprivation can also affect one's mood and ability to tolerate stress, leading to increased irritability.

Considering growing concerns about all types of public health issues and health disparities, it is critical that we restore our reverence for the night and begin to value sleep to reclaim health. In Native communities, we must prioritize revitalizing ancestral sleep practices and spiritual views in the same way we value language preservation and tribal food sovereignty. All people should remember to include sleep as an important component of our total health and wellness. We may be exercising every day, eating healthy meals, spending time outdoors, and incorporating ritual and ceremony, but if we are not sleeping, we simply will not feel or perform our best.

A MEDICINE DREAM
THOSH

> We can imagine the surprise of the first person having an unusual, and perhaps prophetic, dream . . . How eagerly people must have yearned for similar dreams that would guide them in their daily lives!
>
> —*Vine Deloria Jr. (Lakota),* The World We Used to Live In:
> Remembering the Powers of the Medicine Men

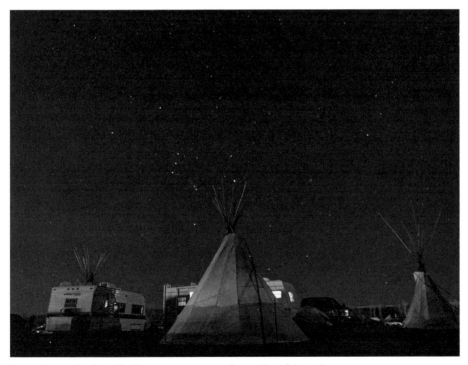

A tipi glows under the night sky as water protectors sleep at Sacred Stone Camp.

It was 2001 and I was in college and living in San Francisco. I didn't have a very healthy sleep pattern in those days. And during that time in my life I was starting to veer off the path that was laid out for me by my family and community, but I didn't yet realize the stakes of such a disconnection from my roots.

Early one morning I was getting ready for school. I had twenty to thirty minutes to spare before I started my usual walk route through the city. Of course, I hadn't gotten a good sleep the night before, so I decided to lie back down on the couch for a few minutes. I lay down with my feet crossed and arms folded across my chest. I was tired but trying not to fall asleep. I closed my eyes and began thinking about everything I needed to do that day. Then I began thinking about which route I was going to take to get to the art college on Lombard. I started visualizing myself walking the route in the city, and then, I don't really know how, I transitioned into the following visual episode.

I was stopped on a street corner and noticed several Native people entering a hotel. They were carrying tote bags and wearing lanyards as if they were attending some type of Native conference. (Many Natives love going to conferences, especially in an exciting city.) So I decided to go in the hotel to see what was going on. I was so excited to see other Native people because I had not yet met many other Native people in San Francisco. I entered the spacious hotel lobby and saw Native people everywhere. The bronze railings, shinning granite floors, and Victorian-style lobby looked very "SF" to me. A short line of people was waiting to check in with their luggage. The lobby was filled with echoes of light chatter among the small groups of visitors. Growing up traveling around the country with the Salt River Youth Council attending Native youth conferences, I found this to be a familiar scene. I felt at home and comfortable.

At this point, I had somehow consciously slipped into a dream-state, but I wasn't yet aware of it. I became very interested in what the conference was about. Searching for the conference registration desk, I walked down a hallway filled with Native folks holding their swag bags. I could vividly smell the faint scent of some type of burning sage and peeked into the room where it was coming from. I saw an elder man who was just finishing smudging off a person.

He looked like a lot of older Native men on reservations in the Southwest or even on the Plains. He was wearing a white straw cowboy hat and a Pendleton vest. He carried a big eagle feather fan. At his feet was a blanket laid out with Native designs, and on it lay a large abalone shell with sage medicine smoldering. Also in the room were a couple of other older Native men dressed the same way, standing side by side talking very quietly. I assumed they were his helpers. A few more conference attendees stood by and quietly visited. The elder man had just finished fanning another person, who quietly thanked him by shaking his hand and nodding his head in acknowledgment.

Then the elder man slowly gestured toward me with his eagle fan, inviting me to come over and get smudged—something we had done often where I grew up. I knew I needed it, so I reluctantly walked over and stood in front of him with my palms facing up in a receiving position, the typical way people stand when they get smudged. He leaned over the smoking medicine and began to repeatedly scoop up some smoke into the eagle wing and then began to fan me. I closed my eyes as I usually do. I literally could feel the wind from the eagle fan blowing against my face. I could smell the familiar scent of the sage. It was all very vivid.

At this point I realized I was no longer in a dream but I was in what we call a "medicine dream." An intense feeling of comfort came over me. It was as if I were being wrapped with a blanket of healing energy. I thought how the feeling was beyond anything that I felt from alcohol and substance use, which were new to me at that time. I felt so comforted that I began to relax all of my muscles—to the point where I began to fall back, but instead of hitting the ground I kept falling. It was as if my consciousness was being shown streaks of light whizzing by to the feeling of comfort and falling. I felt too overwhelmed to handle this and started trying to wake from it. Finally, I abruptly came out of it, my eyes popping wide open, and wondered what had just happened.

I found myself lying exactly as I had lain down a few moments before. As I sat up I realized that I had been passed a message that came to me from a higher source with intentions of guiding me toward a path of healing.

That wasn't the first time I'd had a dream like that, but this one was especially powerful. I knew immediately what this dream was about. I knew that I was falling off the path of a healthy way of life by allowing myself to engage with alcohol and other unhealthy substances and to be influenced by people in the city who had a very different cultural and spiritual outlook from mine. The medicine dream was meant to remind me that consuming mind- and mood-altering substances was not a healthy way of dealing with my stress and that I needed to remember the path that my family and community had laid out for me. I had all of the tools I needed to keep myself well.

This could have been sent to my consciousness by my spirit helpers. Or maybe it was a manifestation of my loved ones who had been praying for me. Maybe some very intuitive and spiritually gifted people from home could sense I was experiencing a hard time, and their prayers came to me in that form. I also believe that our higher selves or spirit consciousness is always connected to the Great Creator, and in some instances Creator is attempting to connect to the unconscious mind when it senses the mind has become out of balance. Usually, the disconnect between the higher spirit consciousness and unconscious mind is a result of trauma or getting too caught up in everyday mundane duties.

In the years after that I had more powerful medicine dreams. Some were obvious and easy to interpret, while others were more ambiguous. But if one isn't able to quickly interpret a dream, it doesn't mean it is a wasted experience. Some dreams and experiences take years, even decades, to make sense of. This notion reflects the understanding that exists in Native culture that because we are only human, it is unfathomable to think that we can understand the immensity of the universe. We don't seek answers in everything. We seek questions.

Once when I as a teen, I was at a ceremonial gathering that began in the middle of a summer night. I was with about thirty men inside an ocotillo structure preparing for a spiritual run. The spiritual leader who was conducting the gathering told us that she'd received a communication from one of our ancestors that each of us should go out and look at one particular star that was shining more brightly than all of the others. She said in her broken English that she didn't know why the ancestor had requested this and gave no further explanation. But she asked us to remember what it looked like, and maybe some years down the line, we would understand what it means.

So one by one, we each went outside of the ocotillo house to gaze up at the western half of the sky. The star was very prominent, making all of the other stars look faint and dim. I stood there for a moment trying hard to figure out what it meant, but nothing came to me. Years later, I asked my dad whether he remembered that, and he replied that he did. "I think of that from time to time," he said, "and I still I don't know what it's about."

Perhaps one of the teachings that came out of that experience was to look to the stars, to look to the sky, to continue to listen and to look to our ancestors for guidance and teaching. Perhaps it was a remembrance to remain humble, to zoom way out and see our place in the universe, and to simply be present.

REMEMBERING HOW TO REST
CHELSEY

> I don't know what being burned out means. I can understand being tired, but after having a peaceful night of rest, everything is okay again. I am always thankful for the things I can still do.
>
> —*Audrey Shenandoah, Onondaga Clan Mother, from* Every Day Is a Good Day:
> Reflections by Contemporary Indigenous Women

Like many people around my age, I remember what life was like without social media, because I had the good fortune of spending my entire childhood without it. I also understand the experience of being in a generation that is totally absorbed in it. I still remember the mystery and excitement of joining Facebook for the first time in 2006, my first year in college. I was hooked right away and used it for the next few years to express my political worldview, to join digital groups, and to create photo memories with my friends. Who knew then that a decade later, I would remove myself from the platform because I experienced bullying, I found it too distracting, and I realized how much of its content was toxic and harmful to my mental health.

Learning to create boundaries and guidelines for myself with social media has been a significant part of my wellness journey in recent years. Experiencing what it's like to get carried away with screen time, and then conversely taking control over this, has made a surprising impact on my ability to rest, relax, and sleep well.

In addition to the more obvious side effects of the growing digital presence in our lives, a surge in screen time has also brought a less obvious burden that is significantly affecting our health: it has taken away so many of our restful moments throughout the day, and it has interfered with our ability to sleep well at night. I can't count the number of nights over the years that I have stayed up late scrolling—whether watching YouTube, checking Instagram, or shopping online. A few years ago, when I began to learn about the negative side effects of screen time, it dawned on me that I had to get serious about limiting myself. No wonder I was getting headaches. No wonder I was cranky during the day. No wonder I was distracted. And no wonder I was having trouble falling asleep.

So many of us don't realize the degree to which electronic devices and screens are interfering with our ability to rest. It's not just about actual sleep, but also about breaks from visual noise and chaotic news. It's interesting that social media is the avenue where "hustle culture" or the glorification of "booked and busy" has become prevalent. I think that we would be better off encouraging one another to take rest when we can and to stop glorifying busyness. Remember to check out of the online world and into the real world. Look up from your phone and look around you. Every day is a gift, and we are harming our health by whiling away the hours online looking to see what other people are doing.

Many of us at this point have experimented with social media fasts or sabbaths. I am no different—in that I have done them, felt great about it, but then ultimately returned to the noise because I use social media to promote my work. My goal now is to eventually divorce my career from my smartphone so that I can stop using that as an excuse. I plan to completely sign off of all forms of social media one day, sooner than later, I hope. I made this decision recently, and I have an "escape plan" brewing. I truly believe that a life without social media will be more restful, more peaceful, and more in line with every other health value that I espouse.

As I have consciously limited my screen time and made a plan to fully exit the virtual world, I know that I am getting closer to living how my ancestors lived—fully present and open to receive teachings in both the real world and the dream world. To be able to rest is a privilege and a gift—one that my parents and grandparents did not come by as frequently as I do. I must work hard and use my gifts, but I should also honor myself and give myself time to simply breathe. This is the life I want my daughters to live, and so, I remember, I owe it to myself to live this life as well.

TAKE ACTION: HOW TO HONOR REST AND SLEEP

Learn
- Through trial and error, observe and take note of how much sleep you need to function optimally. The amount is different for everyone but is typically between seven and ten hours.
- Ask yourself, What does my ideal sleep schedule look like?
- Take note of anything that is currently acting as a barrier to your sleep, such as phone, TV, computer, or other factors.
- Make a plan to prioritize and make time for rest—both "awake" rest and "asleep" rest.
- Consider how you can make your sleeping area more comfortable, peaceful, and serene. This could mean adjusting the temperature, tidying up the room, or rearranging the furniture.

- Seek out the ancestral sleep teachings from your heritage; often, these "legends" or "stories" are a wealth of health knowledge.

Engage
- Remove all electronic devices from the bedroom.
- Learn the "night-light" or "warm-light" settings for laptop, smartphone, and other electronic devices, and turn those on if you have to use devices at night.
- Turn devices off at least one hour before bedtime.
- Implement a whole-family routine for going to bed at night and waking up in the morning.
- Rearrange your schedule to prioritize sleep.
- Read, meditate, do breathing exercises, or engage in other peaceful activities at night in order to prepare for rest.

Optimize
- You are getting the number of hours of sleep every night that is best for your mood and health, and you are prioritizing this in your daily schedule.
- You make time every day to "rest" and engage in ceremony and ritual.
- You have trained your mind to quiet itself when necessary and have realized the importance of integrating these practices into your routine.
- You are exercising regularly during the day so that when it is time to sleep at night, your body is tired and ready to rest.
- You are encouraging and supporting others in your family and workplace to get adequate rest, and you are noticing a reduction in stress for yourself and others.
- You frequently have powerful dreams that guide you in your life, and you have learned to recognize these and listen to them.

INTERSECTION WITH OTHER CIRCLES

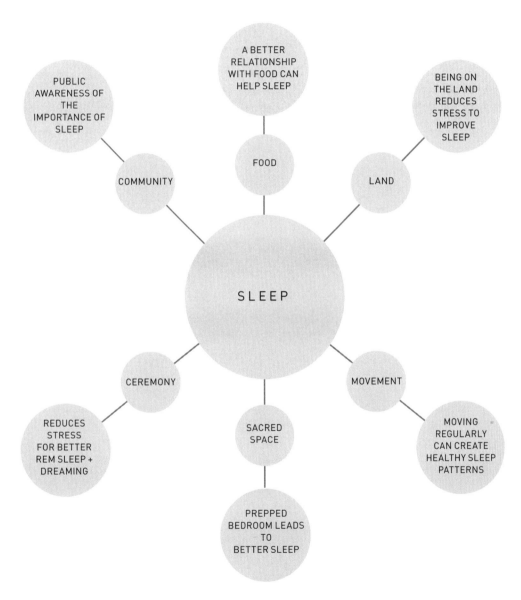

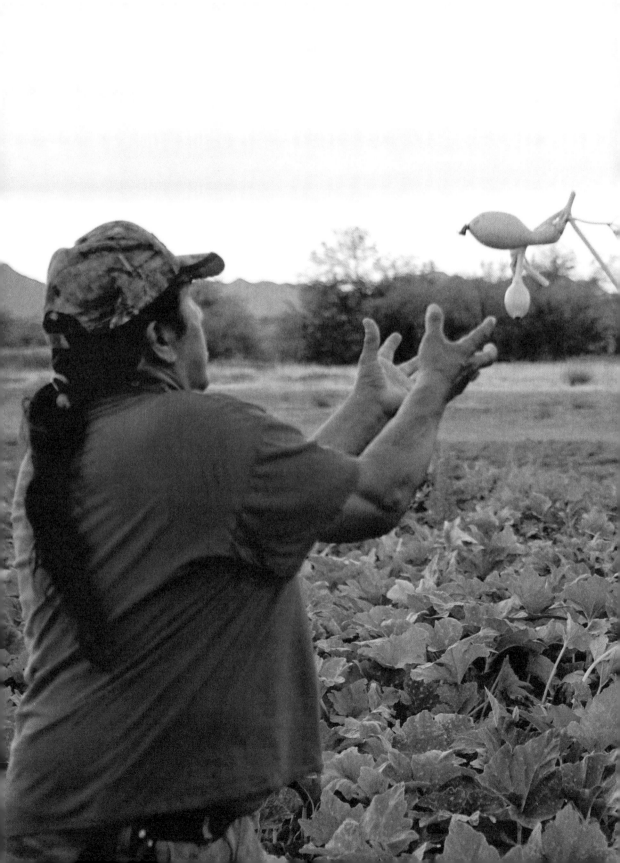

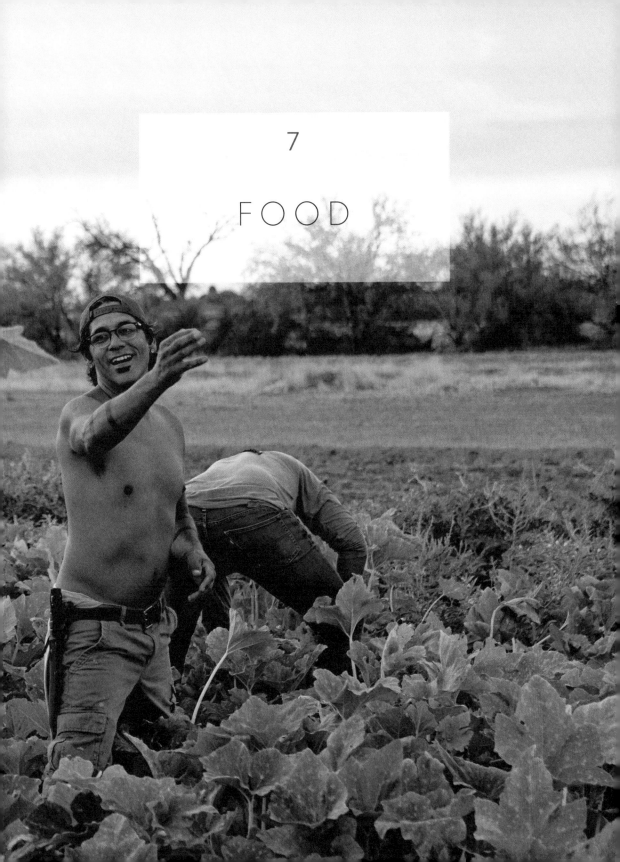

7

FOOD

The world begins at a kitchen table. No matter what, we must eat to live . . . The gifts of earth are brought and prepared, set on the table. So it has been since creation, and it will go on . . . It is here that children are given instructions on what it means to be human.

—Joy Harjo (Mvskoke Creek), from The Women Who Fell from the Sky

REMEMBERING FOOD HISTORY

In the early 1930s, a newlywed couple on the Standing Rock Reservation settled together on a small piece of land on the banks of the Missouri River. Right away, they got into the business of food. They acquired an array of domestic animals, and they grew vegetables. Bit by bit, they saved and bought land, establishing a cattle and bison ranch that would one day span tens of thousands of acres. They opened up the Red and White General Store on the main street of Fort Yates, the reservation's central town. It became a commercial hub for the region, selling everything useful, from clothing to coffee. Eventually, responding to a growing demand for store-bought food due to a rapidly changing reservation economy, they turned the Red and White into the White Buffalo Supervalu, a modern-day grocery store that is still in operation today. This is the story of Thelma and Butch Luger, Chelsey's grandparents.

Meanwhile, another couple on another reservation far away in the Sonoran Desert were also getting into the food business. On the edge of the Salt River Pima–Maricopa Indian Community, when the Phoenix metropolitan area was much less populated and the reservation was still quite rural, a young O'odham couple opened up a small store together. They stocked its shelves with produce that they grew themselves on what land they had left after the homesteading era sold most Pima land off to white settlers. For their community members who no longer had

Previous spread: Richard Blue Cloud Castaneda tosses a squash plant to Tony Collins as they work together to harvest crops in the Collins family field.

access to the resources that allowed them to live off the land, their store provided homegrown O'odham crops like squash, corn, and beans. As other basic goods—such as sugar, flour, and lard—slowly but surely became integrated into the daily lives of O'odham people, they sold those things, too. This is the story of the Collins Market, owned by Cecelia and Ben "Willow" Collins, Thosh's grandparents.

Today we reflect on our grandparents' synchronous stories. Both of these couples saw in their lifetimes great and often devastating change to the land and livelihoods of the people in their communities. They witnessed the shocking effects of urban sprawl and government exploitation of natural resources. They saw their respective rivers—the Missouri and the Salt—get dammed upstream by the Army Corps of Engineers, flooding millions of acres of reservation land to provide power for faraway cities, leaving thousands of Native people with no choice but to stop growing their own food and to rely on canned goods instead. They saw the impacts of government programs, like the Homestead Acts and the Dawes General Allotment Act, that forced a complete shift from Indigenous communal hunting and farming to Western individual landownership. They did their best to meet the food needs of their fellow community members who had been dispossessed and defrauded and were grappling in real time with the fact that they no longer had the economic or political autonomy to feed themselves from the land, as they had done for millennia. The transformation from traditional, to tribal, to family-domestic, to individual capitalistic food culture was not an overnight process, but slowly and surely it seeped its way into Indigenous communities, ultimately causing dire health consequences.

Indigenous people aren't the only group whose health has been negatively affected by the colonization of food. According to the Centers for Disease Control and Prevention, six in ten American adults today suffer from chronic diseases like heart disease, cancer, lung disease, stroke, Alzheimer's, and chronic kidney disease. All of these are rooted in lifestyle factors such as tobacco use, poor nutrition, lack of physical activity, and excessive alcohol use. Four in ten adults are battling two or more of these conditions.[1] In order to begin collective healing, we believe that it is important to acknowledge colonialism, land exploitation, and trauma as the deeper roots of food issues. These massive health problems require systemic change and well-rounded thinking, not fad diets, to address.

Today, people everywhere have come to understand the importance of food for our health, and a growing number are acknowledging that the capitalist infiltration of convenience culture has separated most people from a once-ubiquitous sacred relationship to food. We hope to offer a food approach that rebuilds food-human relationships, while also acknowledging the day-to-day reality of how hard a task this is. There are no quick fixes or overnight solutions. But we have to start somewhere, and we know firsthand that it is possible to be healed and feel restored through certain foods and changes in lifestyle. There are endless healing benefits of developing closer relationships to food and food processes.

We are not here to prescribe a diet or meal plan, as those actions are out of our purview, but we are excited to share with you our method for establishing and maintaining positive relationships to food. May we all invite food back into our lives in a good way, once again understanding its power as a healer, a medicine, and a life-giver.

HOW FOOD HEALS
⊕ Food Medicine Wheel ⊕

SPIRITUAL

Food is a living, life-giving entity. Food and food practices can nourish and fortify us in a spiritual way, as much as in a physically satiating way.

EMOTIONAL

Learning to love and value the healing and nourishing power of food, like our ancestors did, can help to break intergenerational cycles of poor health. Reclaiming autonomy over food processes like harvesting, growing, gathering, and hunting means spending more time on the land, which brings joy, peace, and deep fulfillment.

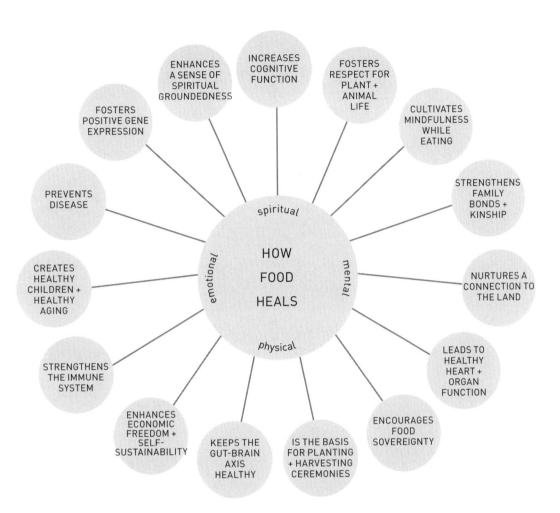

MENTAL

Certain foods have been shown to boost brain function and improve mental clarity, while others can contribute to brain fog and poor concentration. When we integrate healthy, whole foods from the earth like those our ancestors ate, we can think more clearly, work smarter, and communicate better.[2]

PHYSICAL

We are one with our food, Indigenous teachings say, and so in every way, the food that we eat and the way that we go about food processes can impact our health for better or for worse. Food is an integral component of daily personal health care. Know that we all have the power to use food as our medicine.

OUR APPROACH: INDIGENOUS FOODWAYS

Ancestral, paleo dieting is a recent big trend in health circles—one that, ironically, Indigenous communities are often shut out of because they have no access to it or are excluded from the conversation. Although we love learning about the diets of our ancestors, and we know that a strictly precolonial way of eating would almost certainly offer health benefits, we don't push an ancestral diet, because the reality is that this is not a realistic approach for most people. By all means, we support and commend it when people find the resources to take this approach, and indeed we incorporate ancestral foods as often as we can in our personal lives, but we simply can't expect everyone to do so. Since most people don't have the access, support, or skills required to make this complete shift, we developed a food philosophy that we call *Indigenous foodways*. This approach is accessible to all.

In Indigenous foodways there are no rules, restrictions, or limitations—unless you choose to set them yourself. It is a values-based approach that centers gratitude and takes into account factors like accessibility, culture, and budget. It is malleable and adjustable based on different locations, individual needs and preferences, and other variables. Our version of Indigenous eating encourages all people to view food, whether plant or animal, as a life-giving entity to develop a healthy relationship with. It is an approach that constantly evolves. We do not advocate for fad diets because dieting culture has been harmful to so many peoples' health and is especially guilty of excluding and exploiting marginalized communities. However, we respect medical diets and know that these are important for people with certain health conditions who work with their health-care providers to develop food plans that are healing or preventive. In short, Indigenous foodways approaches food and human relationships to food with reverence, patience, dignity, and respect.

The following are a set of Indigenous foodways principles that we encourage you to consider when it comes to food choices and creating your personal food culture. These are not rules, but suggestions to guide you toward an ancestral, holistic approach to food. When possible, Indigenous eating

- Is seasonal
- Is local
- Comes from the land
- Is sustainable and nonexploitative
- Is nutrient dense or nutritionally optimal
- Is culturally significant
- Recognizes a human relationship to food
- Is rooted in gratitude
- Approaches food processes—like hunting, growing, fishing, gathering, cooking, serving, and eating—with reverence and recognizes these methods as inherently spiritual

SEVEN ACTIONS TO STRENGTHEN YOUR RELATIONSHIP TO FOOD

Rooted in our own Indigenous traditions, our family's connection to food culture, and our own experiences feeling restored or depleted by certain ingredients and food processes, we identified seven core actions to reestablish or strengthen a relationship to food. Each of these actions is an important piece of the puzzle in healing our holistic health and approach to diet and foodways. There is something for everyone here. We don't expect all people to do all of these things, but we know that everyone can start today with incorporating at least one of them.

1. Give Thanks

We start with gratitude because this is the action that we all have access to, here and now, no matter who we are, where we live, or what resources are available to us. We can all give thanks.

Begin practicing this even before getting into the weeds of figuring out how to change your diet or any other more complicated aspect of your food practice. Gratitude is central to Indigenous foodways, because we know that without the nourishment of food, we would cease to exist. No matter what food you're eating, whether it be takeout pizza or squash from your garden, you can be spiritually mindful of it. Directing positive thoughts of gratitude toward your food has a positive effect on your entire outlook on life.

We eat every day, so expressing gratitude at mealtime allows you to habitually focus on the good things in life. Studies show positive neurological changes directly associated with gratitude. Expressing gratitude promotes positivity, reduces stress, and even helps a person to be self-motivated and resilient.[3] Our ancestors didn't need such studies to understand why gratitude was central to well-being.

Being present with your food is an important way to demonstrate this gratitude. As you eat, you can think about the hands that helped transport your food on its journey from wherever it began, to wherever it's been, to your table. In some cases taking a deeper look into this process reminds us of the distance that food has traveled and raises important questions regarding the sustainability of our food choices.

Abstain from watching TV or from mindlessly scrolling on electronic devices while you eat. Instead, take some time to examine the flavors and textures of the food and to be good company to the people eating with you. All food was once a living thing, so give thanks for that life that is now nourishing your own life. If you grew, foraged, hunted, or fished the food yourself, you might recollect the hard work and the long process of getting that food to your table. Enjoy the feeling of empowerment that comes from harvesting or cooking your own food.

If you're sharing a meal with family or another group, go around the table and ask everyone to share one thing they are grateful for in general. This is a great

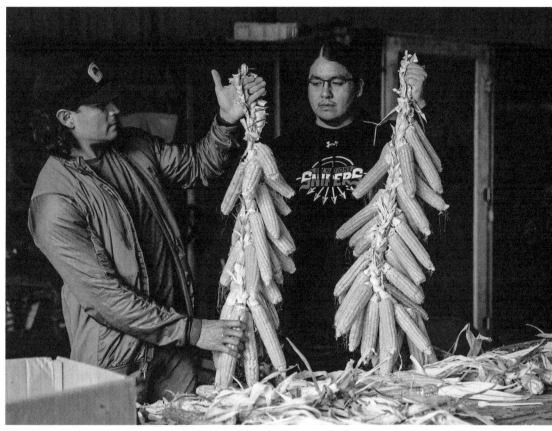

Kaien'kowa:nen Regis Cook (Onandaga) teaches Thosh how to braid Seneca Chief corn.

conversation starter—we learned this from our Native Wellness Institute family members, who always make a point to do this before dinner, no matter how big or small the group. It is especially important for children to see adults expressing their gratitude, as it fosters communication skills and an ability to focus on the good.

2. Hunt and Fish

For centuries, Indigenous people have relied on hunting and fishing, in many cases for the bulk of the calories and nutrients that they needed to survive and be strong. The notion that one life thrives by the expiration of another is one of the most fascinating paradoxes of our existence as human beings. Hunting and fishing, at their core, are about acquiring protein and fat from sustainable animal sources, in the most ethical way.

In today's culture, many people view hunting as cruel or unnecessary. We don't see it that way. We recognize that whether plant or animal, we must rely on others' lives to survive. It is normal, not harmful. Only overexploitation and the continued destruction of animal habitats are harmful. But if done responsibly, hunting and fishing can be healthful, intimate, and humane. Hunting one's own meat also provides one with the most thorough understanding of its value. Truly, it fosters a relationship between the hunter and the hunted.

The process of hunting and fishing is not available or of interest to everyone today, but for those who would like to begin, proper preparation starts with the mind. It is important to have the best intentions in your heart and mind when intending to take a life to feed your own. Honor and reverence for the animals being hunted, fished, and farmed should be at the forefront. The "slow-food" culture of hunting, foraging, and gardening can teach much about how sacred food is. Having a hand in every step of the process offers you a true understanding of where food comes from and how much time, effort, and care go into the journey to our tables.

If you are learning to hunt, it is very important to have a mentor with years of experience who can teach you about the process. Hunting is a skill. Taking a hunters' education course is helpful. After a shift in mindset, you must find out which species are available for you to hunt or fish. Only hunt if you are confident you can make use of the whole animal so that its life will not go in vain. Learn the different techniques of hunting, and continue to hone the craft because a merciful death of an animal is at stake and is dependent on you making an ethical kill to prevent undue pain and suffering to the animal.

Trophy hunting has never been the Indigenous way. For us, hunting is a ceremony, and we spend our lives honoring, praying for, and fostering good environments for the animals who sacrifice so that we may live.

3. Forage

Foraging wild plant food on the land is something almost everyone can do. Every region of Mother Earth offers something unique, and our Indigenous ancestors took full advantage of this since it was one of their core means of food acquisition.

As the Earth moves around the sun, the land changes with the seasons, bringing different foods to the land and inviting us to partake in the slow-foods culture. Like hunting, fishing, and gardening, foraging is a way to align ourselves with the seasons and the spirit of the land we're living upon. As we consume local, wild, and slow foods, we are inviting the land to be integrated with our bodies. The microbiome both in our guts and on our bodies changes the more we engage with and consume wild foods.

From the labor of navigating the land to picking the foods and enduring longer periods of times to cure and process that food, we learn a new kind of appreciation for food and the way of life that our ancestors lived in order for us to be here today. We being to understand why food was highly revered and why our people found it necessary to have ceremonies to honor the coming of the foods on the land. We're reminded of where it all started and what it truly means to be a human being. When we're keeping a good heart and mind and staying present in the process, we begin to feel that the plant nations put new teachings in our consciousness. They teach us new ways to care for them, new ways to process and prepare them for our nourishment. When we abstain from the desire to take pictures and videos of the foraging process, we experience a sense of peacefulness. We begin to take notice of the land and grow a new sense of appreciation for and feeling of connectedness.

Even if you're able to harvest only one plant per year or if you're able to get only a handful of food to include along with the rest of your store-bought food, it's still a good thing to do.

4. Grow

Much like foraging, growing food can be done almost anywhere and by anyone. No matter how large or small the scale, growing food is a deeply spiritual process that can transform your perspective on life. Some say that a person should learn to grow food before they have children, because it will prepare that person to devote time, energy, patience, attention, and effort into another life. If you have access to land, on your own property or in a community garden, you may grow larger crops, like squash, potatoes, or corn. If you have access to just a balcony or windowsill, you may grow smaller plants, like herbs, peppers, or greens.

Just as animal life is honored, plant life should be honored too. If you decide to grow food, you should commit to the seeds that you plant and don't neglect them before they produce. So much of life today is dependent on instant satisfaction. Growing will shift your mindset toward the joys of long-term commitment and steady care. Growing food is a mutually beneficial relationship between human and plant life that will bring healing to anyone who commits to it.

5. Shop

As much as we love to advocate for food sovereignty and sustainability through hunting, fishing, foraging, and gardening, most people today, ourselves included, must rely on buying food from grocery stores or other markets. We believe it is important to learn to navigate the grocery store efficiently. Throughout our travels and work in Native Country, many people have expressed feeling overwhelmed by the endless aisles and options available in grocery stores. Generally, the outer perimeter of the store consists of produce and meats, so we want to start there because these are the nutrient-dense base items that make the bulk of our meals. Dried goods, like beans or grains, are affordable and are also often found near the produce. In the aisles, we then get our condiments such as cooking oils or seasonings, and whatever packaged foods we might need. We also recommend finding a grocery store that you enjoy and sticking with it. The better you know your store, the easier and more intuitive your shopping experience will become.

6. Cook

Cooking is one of the things that makes us human. Cooking is like a ceremony. Elders always tell us that we must have a good mind and heart when we're cooking food for others, because someone is going to eat that food and ingest whatever we put into it, ingredients and emotions. Feeding someone food to nourish their health is one of the most loving things you can do for a person. In our cultures we have a tradition of feasting. Native families find honor in being able to invite people into their homes to feed them. All across the United States and Canada we've had the wonderful opportunity of being invited into peoples' homes to eat the food they have lovingly prepared for us. These meals are always accompanied by good talks about healing, wellness, and food culture. We must restore the importance of cooking once again, rather than relying on ordering in or fast food.

Getting comfortable with cooking is an empowering way to take control of our health. Through cooking, we develop a relationship to each ingredient we use, from spices to produce, understanding how they work in relation to other foods. It is also a good activity to do with children because it helps them feel included and productive. Children are born to be helpers. We can strengthen our family relationships by processing food, shopping, and cooking together to sit down and eat mindfully.

To keep things exciting, experiment with different modes of cooking. Try old techniques such as cooking outside or pitting meat in the ground. But explore the new technologies of cooking too. In our home we use an instant pot almost daily for its ability to cook Indigenous beans and Ojibwe wild rice quickly. Find and get familiar with the core, staple tools or accessories that assist you with cooking. For us, it's our cast iron pans, our wooden spatula and spoon, our butcher block cutting board, and a good sharp knife or two.

Recipes can be used as reference points to start learning to cook. We can view them as flexible templates rather than rigid guidelines that we must follow. The goal is to eventually become an intuitive cook. You will cook more quickly and more often once you develop a skill for modifying, substituting, and making a variety of meals with an array of ingredients on hand. In our situation, when we pick foods from the land or select them from the grocery store, we don't always know exactly how we're going to work them into a meal. But we are confident we can find a use for them.

People have told us that they run out of recipes, or don't know any, so they let the food in their fridge go to waste and end up eating out instead. It definitely is a learning process that will require some time and consistency. Keep at it, prepare to fail from time to time (we still do), enjoy the experimenting process, and don't give up.

7. Breastfeed or Support Feeding Freedom

We believe that all mothers and parents should have the freedom to feed their infants however they want and that all mothers and parents should be given the space, time, and respect that is necessary to feed comfortably. Whether using formula, breastfeeding on demand, pumping breast milk, or anything else that works, it is important that a baby is fed on the caretaker's terms.

In Indigenous food culture, we talk about breastfeeding as a spiritual, ancestral process that is sacred to us. In Western society, because of the imposition of patriarchy and the policing of women's bodies, breastfeeding is still looked down upon by many. Women are expected to cover up in public if they are breastfeeding, they are made to feel uncomfortable, and workplaces are not giving adequate maternity leave so that feeding can be done on demand.

Breastfeeding is a powerful process that can offer myriad benefits to mothers and babies, including nurturing emotional well-being, preventing postpartum depression, contributing to adequate nutrition, supporting the immune system, preventing cancer, and more. All people, whether parents or not, should recognize that demanding space and respect for women to feed their babies however they choose is paramount to maternal health, infant health, and collective well-being.

THE EVOLUTION OF
MY PERSONAL FOOD CULTURE
CHELSEY

My stepdad loves to remind me that when I was in kindergarten, I used to proudly tell everyone that I wanted to be a Schwan Man when I grew up. Schwan's food delivery was a service that came by our house once a week in the 1990s, selling pizzas, chocolate chip ice cream, and other frozen foods. I didn't always grow up with a deep and spiritual connection to food. Far from it. I actually preferred anything frozen, packaged, or boxed, because those foods seemed more normal to me than anything fresh from a field or a hunt, like my ancestors would have eaten. I remember that when we did have fresh, home-cooked meals for dinner, like a roast with veggies, I would pass my carrots under the table to my sister Liz because I could not stand to eat them. I was also the least likely of all of my sisters to lend a hand in the kitchen or to show any interest in cooking.

Growing up, I also regularly saw and ate culturally specific Native American foods, though usually not ancestral. I'm talking about rez foods. At my grandma and grandpa Herman's house in Turtle Mountain, they often cooked "bullets and bangs" (soup and frybread) or Indian tacos. I loved commodity cheese sandwiches on white bread, and I equally loved commodity cereal. While foods like this are certainly not precolonial, they are culturally significant, and I think that understanding their prevalence on Native reservations helps to paint a picture of the reality of Indigenous food culture today. When I was a kid, I would see truly "traditional foods," like *was'na* (dried bison meat with dried, ground chokecherries) or *tinpsila* (wild turnips), about once or twice a year when I went to ceremonies or cultural gatherings with my dad.

My food journey has come a long way. When I was in my twenties in college, I started to notice how a well-rounded meal gave me more energy to study and think more clearly, and a few years later, I started to learn about how food has always been sacred to my ancestors. Now, we regularly integrate Indigenous foods into our meals, and we cook every day with whole, nourishing ingredients that we buy at the grocery store. I drink water and unsweetened tea rather than the Dr. Pepper or fruit juice I grew up with. I avoid or limit foods that my body does not respond well to, like dairy and gluten, and I am always making an effort to quell my sugar addiction. I love when we get to eat venison that my husband has hunted or squash that we have grown in our family field, and I am happy that my kids recognize this as a normal part of life. I am glad to now be a part of the tribal food sovereignty conversation, and to have reclaimed a relationship to food, not only because it keeps me physically healthy and strong, but because it nourishes my spirit.

I approach the topic of food with patience and understanding because of my lived experiences. I know the hard work it takes to relearn and undo unhealthy lifestyle habits that have become cultural norms. I know the history of colonialism and systemic injustices Indigenous peoples and other groups have experienced that have made food culture so complicated in the first place. I see a lot of fear-mongering in wellness circles today, which I believe is an unhelpful tactic that pushes people farther away from developing a safe and healthy relationship to food. Pushing fad diets and making overblown statements like "anything packaged is bad for you" or "preservatives will make you sick" can make people feel ashamed and afraid to ask questions or learn more. Certainly, we can acknowledge that the nutritional composition of foods can vary depending on how they are packaged and prepared, and we can encourage critical thinking on the topic. But making sweeping statements that may exclude groups of people is unhelpful. So like all things in health, we must be delicate, we must be compassionate, and we must be kind when talking about food.

I recently spoke at a wellness gathering with participants from all over the world. I met a woman from Italy who told me a good story on this topic. She said that when she first began her wellness journey and was learning a lot about food, she told her grandmother that they should no longer eat pasta and that she was definitely not going to eat any carbs after three o'clock in the afternoon. Her grandmother laughed and shrugged it off. The woman later realized how little this made sense. "I'm doing all of this in the name of seeking *purity*," she said, "but what is more pure than the love that my grandmother puts into the food she makes for me? Her food is how she shows her love." In this woman's case, is it wrong to rethink dietary choices? No. But she realized that she can do so in balance, without dismissing her special heritage foods. Sometimes food nourishes in ways other than nutrient density, and we can include that knowledge while also setting guidelines that make sense for our health.

What has truly motivated me to reclaim Indigenous foods, and to approach eating healthier, has not been the shameful messaging from diet culture, or the body image comparisons from mainstream media, or even the colorful messaging from health influencers. What really got me fired up about food was understanding its interconnectedness with social justice, community well-being, and intergenerational healing. From there, I began the process of experimenting with recipes, learning to cook, learning to grow, taking an interest in hunting, learning about the different regions and styles of Indigenous cuisine, and figuring out how I can integrate those things, in a realistic way, into life for me and my kids. No amount of pressure or shaming can motivate people into a sustainable, healthy way of life. We have to go deeper than that, and we have to lead with compassion.

RECLAIMING O'ODHAM FOOD CULTURE
THOSH

There is a sentence that has followed me and bothered me my entire life: "Pimas (the government term for O'odham) have the highest rates of type 2 diabetes in the world." I grew up hearing people say this, and I still come across this statistic all the time, commonly cited in all types of health books and resources today. When I was a kid, I heard the word "diabetes" so often that I thought it was a word in the O'odham language!

For me, learning about and reclaiming a connection to land and original Indigenous foodways is not just about my personal health, but about reclaiming family

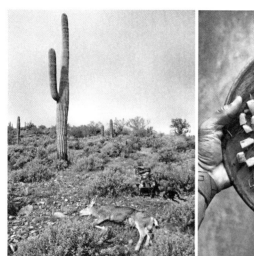 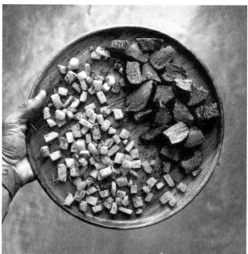 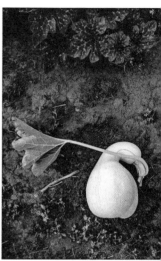

A field-to-table meal, entirely hand-harvested with song, ceremony, love, and gratitude by Thosh Collins and family. Left: Mule deer buck harvested on the Salt River Reservation. Center: The final product, a plate of seared squash with rosemary and slices of venison. Right: O'odham ha:l *(squash) from the Collins family field.*

and community health as well. The big-picture story of my nation shows something more: that poor health and depressing statistics are relatively recent, and we have a much richer, ancient history of good health and physically thriving people. I wish the general public knew our complete story and that our own people had the freedom to stop internalizing these negative statistics about diabetes. That part of our story has become too prevalent, and I've seen what happens when we begin to accept it as our fate. I hope that by offering my perspective, I can help to humanize statistics like this, inviting others to understand that reclaiming a spiritual, symbiotic relationship to food is not just an interesting hobby, but a life-saving process that impacts spiritual life, family life, and nationhood.

As a teen, I remember our cultural and ceremonial leaders discussing a notable drop-off in participation at our spiritual runs and other ceremonies. We talked about all the possible reasons why this could be—lack of family support, distractions from nearby city life, or people getting caught up in drugs and alcohol.

The decreased participation in spiritual life was reflected in other public health statistics collected by the tribe. Some things that we didn't bring up were historical trauma, environmental degradation, and colonialism. But these, I've since learned, are the true root causes of declining community and individual health.

When our river was dammed, our people were forced to accept the American way of individual landownership, and our traditional agricultural system became no longer economically viable, we simultaneously started to eat, shop, and live the American way, which led to what we're seeing today: an increase in diabetes, addiction, domestic violence, gang activity, and economic inequity. Again, there is nothing inherently, biologically, or culturally wrong with us as people— although some still suggest this. This condition of poor health has been imposed upon us. We have to work hard to reclaim the connection to food that we once had, which kept us healthy and thriving for thousands of years.

For a long time, knowing how bad diabetes and other diseases were in my community, I got frustrated when I saw sugary drinks and heavy foods that lacked nutrients being served at all of our community gatherings. I had a vendetta against frybread and used to take to social media to criticize anyone who made a "choice" to serve such foods to our people. Eventually, I realized it was wrong to have such a judgmental attitude. I still regret making comments in person and online that might have made people feel insecure about their lack of knowledge about healthy living. So I made it a point to be understanding of people's conception of healthy food and be more gentle about offering perspectives about creating a healthy connection to food. I now know that food addiction and lifestyle diseases are often manifestations of trauma. Not everyone is fortunate enough to have access to food literacy or to experience nourishing home-cooked meals during their upbringing.

Growing up, I tried our original O'odham foods only occasionally, mostly at ceremonies. When I returned to Arizona in my early thirties, my younger brother Amson was working for the cultural resource department and became very involved with learning about and reclaiming the seasonal foraging and farming of O'odham foods, such as *hun*, *bav*, and *ha:l* (corn, beans, and squash). Although he and I had already been hunting growing up, learning to forage and grow foods from the land really strengthened our connection to food. We decided to get our field back in shape and ready to grow food again.

A few years before that my dad planted melons, squash, beans, and varieties of peppers and chiles. Decades before him, his *ba:b* (maternal grandfather) grew alfalfa, corn, squash, and melons. So we were proud to carry on the tradition of growing food on our land. I learned a great deal from elders and other experienced community people about teachings and practices around O'odham foods.

In particular I enjoyed learning about the nutritional values of O'odham foods. Many of them contain nutrients and trace minerals that are lacking in the standard American diet that our people were forced to adopt. For example, the *s-tota bav* (white tepary bean), *huñ* (sixty-day corn), and *ha:l* are diabetic friendly, since they are complex carbohydrates that are high in fiber and provide more sustainable energy than other common carbohydrate sources. Harvesting the *hanam* (buckhorn cholla cactus buds) is a process I have grown to especially love. According to the Tohono O'odham Community Action group, two tablespoons of dried cholla cactus buds provide as much calcium as a glass of milk. Yet that glass of milk has more than a hundred calories while *hanam* has only twenty-eight. The buds contain a gel-like substance that slows down the absorption rate of sugar into the blood.[4]

Like growing, hunting, or harvesting anything else in the original way, preparing *hanam* is a lengthy process that takes much more time and energy than picking something up at a restaurant or store. But experiencing the slow-food culture has been a joy that changed my view of how important original foodways are, not only for our physical health but also for our sense of belonging to the land and connecting to those we are working with. Similarly, the ceremonial aspect of food culture helped me to understand the health implications of food more completely. Food goes beyond just nutritional value. It is a physical expression of how we as humans are vulnerable in and dependent on the natural world. That is the core of our spiritual relationship to food. Understanding this, my entire outlook on food changed forever.

The more I learned about O'odham and other Indigenous foodways, the more profoundly it began to dawn on me how urgent it is to prioritize the reclamation of our original healthy foodways and lifestyles to prevent the onset of modern diseases and the reality of day-to-day suffering that such diseases cause. I believe that this is a lesson those in mainstream culture can learn from as well, as a disconnection from real food is equally if not more prevalent outside of Indigenous communities.

Now, when we have community gatherings, or when I am asked to speak with children, I try to include all of this information, reminding people that our foodways, community health, movement practices, connection to land, and every other aspect of health—indeed, the Seven Circles of this book—are interconnected. I encourage people to seek out healthier options for food and drink rather than the usual frybread, potato salad, and heavily refried beans, and I proactively offer ideas as to what these options could be. Many other O'odham people are also invested in health reclamation, and I am so excited and encouraged that we are beginning to see greater attention and awareness to creating diabetic-friendly spaces within our cultural settings.

As a father and husband, I realize how critical it is to foster a connection to land and food for my daughters. I want this to be the norm for them, their friends, and the rising generations of O'odham youth. Including our baby girls in harvesting, growing, and hunting has been a challenging but fun process for me and Chelsey. I'll never forget our first little family hunt when we went out in search of *kokji* (javelina), a piglike animal that is native to our area. O'odham have been hunting *kokji* for centuries. Amidst the foothills of Red Mountain on the rez, with Alo on my back in a child carrier and Westyn in a baby carrier on Chelsey trailing behind us, I spotted one about two hundred yards away. Careful not to spook it by being too loud, or to let it track our scent, we quietly approached it until it settled under a palo verde tree. When ready, my arrow flew straight and true. The *kokji* dropped where it was standing and expired not long after, making it a clean and ethical kill. I was so excited to be able to do that all with Alo on my back, just like our people might have done in the old days.

I felt proud to fulfill my philosophy of being "well for culture," and I was proud of Alo too. Her silence and calmness allowed me to be successful in my shot. I talked to her carefully about the life and death of the animal, and included her as I prayed in gratitude for its sacrifice. Her serious disposition showed that she understood. On the way home, we recounted the experience so she could further process what she had witnessed. Hunting and eating meat perfectly exemplifies what I call the most fascinating paradox of our existence: in order for one life to be nourished, the life of others must end in some way and at some time. Since I was young, my father always honored the life of the animal in a ceremonial way. I continue to do that myself. Within the words of thanks I state my intention of how I and my family will use the animal for our nourishment. I ask it to be with me in spirit and help guide me in life.

The connection we foster between ourselves and our food is a lifelong quest. Currently, we're not nearly at the level we'd like to be when it comes to growing, foraging, and hunting for our food. But with every generation and passing season we become stronger and closer to the connection our Indigenous ancestors once had.

HOW WE EAT IN OUR HOME

The definition of Indigenous foodways is constantly evolving, given how our cultures are now intersecting with and a part of mainstream society in many ways. Every family has the right to define the best way for them to eat: culturally, spiritually, economically, and nutritionally. This will look very different from family to family, even within a particular community.

As mentioned, we do not offer specific nutritional advice, nor do we wish to cause any confusion. However, you're probably wondering what we eat and how we apply Indigenous eating to our own lives. So we'll tell you what we do. Please keep in mind that this is our personal method, not a recommendation.

Interestingly, we eat very similarly to how our grandparents ate during the transformative reservation era we mentioned at the beginning of this chapter.

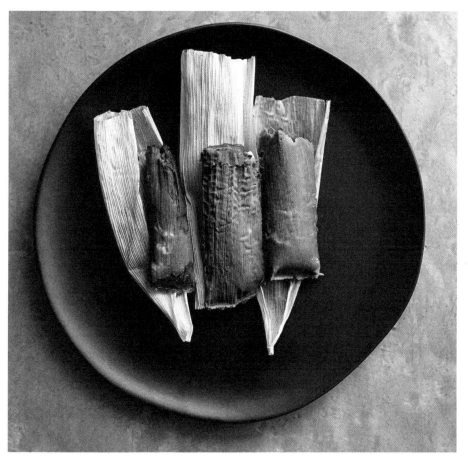

Tamales, a well-known and widely loved Indigenous food, prepared with blue corn masa and venison from one of Thosh's hunts. Made by Carmen Guerrero.

Like them, we are at a crossroads of a domestic, self-sustained food culture—one that relies on industry and capitalism. Simple meats, carbs, and vegetables seasoned with salt and pepper often comprise the bulk of our meals. We have days when we eat out and get pizza, and we often snack on popcorn, chips, and other treats. But for the most part, we try to stay mindful of and careful about our choices, from a nutritional standpoint.

We take a hybridized approach to our own food culture. We come from different Indigenous nations in our small household, and so we eat a mix of Indigenous and non-Indigenous foods. We hunt, forage, fish, grow, and gather when we can, but we also regularly shop at the grocery store. On any given night, our plate will be a mix of Indigenous and conventional foods. We use typical condiments like olive oil, sauces, and seasonings and have our fair share of snack foods that we like to indulge in from time to time. Sometimes we order from online sustainable, ethical, and tribally owned sources Indigenous foods that are hard to come by or that are not local to us, like bison or wild rice. When we are able to include local, self-harvested foods in our meals, we recognize the privilege in this, and we feel grateful for the ability to stay connected to the land.

In the future we aim to be even more self-sustainable than we are now. If we can get to a place where we are growing/hunting/gathering at least 50 percent of our food, and thus relying less on the grocery store, we will be very happy. That scenario would be great progress. Right now, we're slowly getting there.

Even as a Native family who is passionate about health and food sovereignty, we can't just snap our fingers and overnight live that lifestyle. We don't have complete access to our original foods for a number of reasons. However, eating with Indigenous values in mind is something we can do every time we eat, no matter if the food we're eating is processed or something we harvested ourselves.

We estimate proper food portions using our hands—a method we learned from our oral tradition and a technique people from many cultures have used for generations. Typically, for meat and protein, it is recommended that you eat a piece that can fit in the palm of your hand. For carbohydrates, it's anywhere from one to two closed-fist-size portions, depending on your needs. For fats and oils, we measure with the width and length of our index finger.

Before the industrial food era, eating too much food at once was discouraged because survival depended on food rationing. In Thosh's community, elders have told stories about times when food was plentiful, and in one day, people generally ate an amount of food that could fit in both hands cupped together. In the winter when food was scarce, they ate only about one handful per day, or sometimes they would fast. On a typical day, they would wait six to eight hours between each meal because they were busy working. There was not much time, or food, to be snacking throughout the day. Today people call this "intermittent fasting" or "time-restricted eating" to better control caloric intake. But these trends reflect the way people have been eating for generations. We live today in an age of plenty, so we can learn from these stories as they provide insight into portion sizes and Indigenous foodways.

Our personal food culture also requires us to understand how much protein, fat, carbohydrates, and fiber our bodies require. This will vary from person to person and also depends on one's goals or needs for athletic performance, preventive health care, and other factors. Our ancestors understood very well that different foods provide different nutrients for their bodies, so the concept of targeting macronutrients and micronutrients is not entirely new. Like all other aspects of "eating healthy," it is a tradition we are continuing.

We'd like to emphasize that our food culture and choices change seasonally, and we are always making tweaks or adjustments depending on how active we have been, where we are going, what we are doing, whether we are cooking for others, what our kids want to eat, and more. We try to be mindful and to make nourishing choices, while also being flexible. Above all, we remain grateful for our food.

THE MEAT CONVERSATION

The Indigenous perspective on the "anti-meat narrative" is almost never included in the conversation, and it is unique. There is a false narrative that members of Native communities who eat meat, hunt, and fish are active participants in harmful and unsustainable practices. This is not accurate, however. Native communities have been conservators of animal life for thousands of years and still maintain sacred relationships, rooted in gratitude and reciprocity, with the wildlife populations that they hunt and fish. There is a false veil of morality behind this critique and an inherent ignorance of how important eating meat, hunting, and fishing are to us from a nutritional standpoint, as well as being our political right and critical to our cultural continuity and spiritual well-being.

Family, individual, or tribal hunting and fishing are not the root causes of harm to wildlife populations and habitats. Mass colonial land grabs, urban sprawl, corporate agriculture, dams, deforestation, and commercialized food systems are the root and ongoing causes of decimated animal populations. Many people who eat vegan or plant-based diets get their food from corporate farms, which occupy swaths of land that continue to displace animal populations. These acres of monoculture occupy space where diverse wildlife, diverse ecosystems, and indeed diverse tribal nations once thrived. Part of an Indigenous perspective on food and land is an understanding of give and take, of restraint within consumption. So while there have been important evolving conversations about food production, ethics, and sustainability, there have also been holes in the conversation that an Indigenous perspective can help fill. The claim that any diet is "harm-free" and "does not take life" is harmfully binary, ignorant of nuance, and dismissive of colonial history.

We have yet to hear a vegan outline the important context of the buffalo genocide, for example. In the 1600s, as many as sixty million buffalo roamed North America on expansive, biodiverse grasslands. Indigenous people hunted these buffalo with restraint, honoring them as our sacred relatives who provided food and shelter, using every single piece of their bodies for something useful. As white settlers continued to encroach during the 1800s, the federal government initiated a program that paid hunters for every buffalo life taken, with the goal of destroying the Native food supply, livelihood, and economy. This vicious tactic worked. By the 1880s, wild buffalo were nearly extinct. Similar stories of deliberate wildlife extinction by white settlers, to harm Native populations, can be found across the world—whether it be salmon, whales, or other animals that Native people maintained good relationships with. These ties were all but severed by settler colonialism. It is a miracle that Native people have been able to maintain any semblance of traditional hunting and fishing culture at all, and where we have, we should be supported.

With this in mind, perhaps we can think more critically about the anti-meat narrative. Rather than accepting a black-and-white, cut-and-dried solution at face value, we need to think about the bigger picture. Perhaps instead of telling all people, regardless of background or history, to stop eating meat, one could initiate a campaign to restore grasslands for bison or to further educate people about the buffalo genocide. To accept the notion that all humans must stop eating meat in order to help sustain the environment is to accept as unequivocal truth the belief that the extinction of animal biodiversity and the destruction of the earth itself are inevitable. To say "not eating meat is the best way to do your part for the environment" is an avenue to give ourselves a pat on the back without thinking realistically about the complexity of the issue. It also dismisses the nutritional needs of many Indigenous communities.

Human beings have evolved in reciprocity with diverse animal and plant life. Many of us still rely on meat today. The imposition of a plant-based narrative from a standpoint of moral superiority is inherently anti-Indigenous.

FIRST FOOD CEREMONY

Before our kids were born, we learned that one of our responsibilities as parents is to begin to foster their connection to the land, our culture, and our original foodways. When we were pregnant, we spent a lot of time outside working in our field, digging in the dirt with bare feet and bare hands, and discussing the significance of what it means to help life grow. We ate Indigenous foods and other nourishing foods that come from the earth as often as possible so that even from within the womb, our daughters would begin to be nourished by them.

There is a teaching that says anyone who wants to be a parent should learn how to grow corn first, because it requires a similar level of love, attention, consistency, and patience. By growing food, we began to learn how to raise children. Later in the pregnancy, during the warm fall and into the winter, spending time outside, moving and caring for plants, kept our minds and hearts in the right place.

Alo's birth was hard and long. She was more than two weeks past due. We were in the hospital for seven days, and she eventually had to arrive via emergency C-section. Our small victory was that she started breastfeeding right away, making that journey easier than we had expected. When spring planting came around, we strapped her in the baby wrap carrier and took her with us. We joined the rest of our family as we prayed for the health of the plants and for the health of one another, especially our brand new baby. As we started the planting process, we sang songs, we prayed over the seeds, and when we were ready to put the seeds in the ground, everyone smiled and watched as we knelt down and used Alo's little foot to cover the first seed with dirt.

Several months later, when it came time for her to try solid food for the first time, we set up an outdoor feast next to the field, not far from where her placenta had been buried a few days after she was born. We harvested a squash that she had helped to plant. By then it had grown to full size. Alongside our family, we witnessed her first tasting of food. We felt so grateful that we were able to feed her an O'odham squash that came from seeds that have been passed down her paternal bloodline for generations. In this way, we rooted her in the land by nourishing her with her ancestors' foods. As she grew older, however, she suffered from a feeding disorder, which prevented her from learning to eat in line with the typical developmental timeline. She is still learning to eat today. Watching her go through this, witnessing her bravery and determination, we have learned to cherish food and eating in ways we never otherwise would have understood.

A few years later, we approached our daughter Westyn's first food ceremony in a slightly different way, but with the same intention. In order to provide balance, to honor our relationships to animal life (as we already honored our plant relatives during Alo's ceremony), we decided that Westyn's first food would be from an animal. We prepared her bone broth that came from one of the deer that Thosh had hunted before she was born. During Alo's ceremony, we had focused on our tradition of growing and agriculture, while for Westyn's ceremony, we focused on our tradition of hunting.

The ceremonies are important, and equally important are the stories that go along with them. For years to come, we will make a point of telling our daughters about their first food ceremonies. With care, we will explain the meaning behind

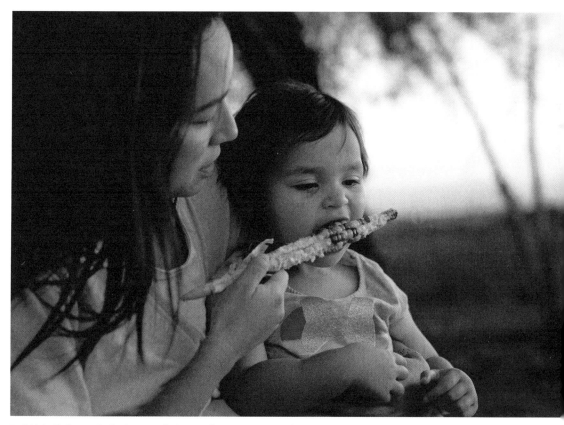

In 2014, Chelsey and Thosh were gifted seeds of this Arikara corn from seed keepers in the Shakopee-Mdewakanton Dakota Community, who were previously gifted them from Arikara people in North Dakota. In 2018, they grew the corn in the Collins family field. Here, Alo enjoys a taste after it was freshly picked and roasted on an outdoor fire. Indigenous seed exchanges remain an important aspect of traditional foodways and tribal food sovereignty.

them; tell them why we chose each food, which were local to the land and historically significant; and pass on the teachings of respecting plant and animal life that are associated with them. As parents, we find it empowering to continue the food culture that our ancestors carried on for thousands of years. We see this culture as a means of connecting our children directly to their ancestors, allowing them to taste, experience, and respect food in the same way that their people always have. In this way, they will understand who they are as human beings, they will become affirmed in their identity, and they will always be connected to the land. Interestingly, Alo continues to gravitate toward corn tortillas and tomato soup, while Westyn strongly prefers bites of medium-rare steak.

The ways that we did these first food ceremonies are not necessarily widely taught in either of our nations, nor did we do them the way our ancestors did for thousands of years. But as an intertribal family who are committed to reclaiming ancestral parenting practices, we came up with the ideas for how we would do these ceremonies while discussing the reverence that our people have always had for land and food. We often discuss the various ways that we, as parents, can root our daughters in good health in sustainable ways.

We believe that our ancestors would have supported our version of a first food ceremony for our family. We encourage all people to consider these important milestones in a child's life as an opportunity for expressing story, reverence, and gratitude alongside your children.

TAKE ACTION:
HOW TO STRENGTHEN
YOUR RELATIONSHIP TO FOOD

Because the food circle is very complex, we have broken it down into further categories within Learn, Engage, and Optimize:

- Ancestral Foodways
- Nutrition/Physical Health
- Everyday Lifestyle Integration/Enjoyment

Learn
- Ancestral Foodways

- Which foods are meaningful to you, culturally significant to your heritage, and important for you to keep within your food culture?
- Learn the history of your people's original foods (creation story).
- Learn about the spiritual protocols, prayers, and songs associated with the respectful planting and harvesting of foods (animal and agriculture).
- Learn the names of the foods in your Indigenous language.
- Are you interested in foraging, hunting, fishing, and gardening? Does your land support this lifestyle to any degree, even if only on a small scale?
- Do you have access to mentors with knowledge about these food systems? Learn who they are and find out how you can respectfully shadow them or hire them to teach you.
- Are any tribal programs available in your community offering or facilitating ancestral foodways?—such as community gardens, hunting education, ranches that provide buffalo meat, etc.
- For dietitians, diabetes educators, and health advocates who work in tribal communities: hold yourself accountable for learning environmental history, traditional foodways, and the degree to which loss of access to these things has impacted the health of your clientele's health. Make an effort to reintegrate this information.
- Nutrition/Physical Health
  - What are your health concerns, medical requirements, and nutritional needs (such as dietary restrictions)?
  - What amount and type of foods are suitably nourishing in line with your level of physical activity?
  - Learn about different options for monitoring your food intake (for example, calorie counting, macronutrient measurements, or hand portion sizes).
  - Where are the grocery stores, markets, and other resources in your area that you can consistently access for procuring food?
  - How can you center food more closely to the core of your day-to-day priorities?
  - Begin to teach yourself the basics about nutritional biochemistry. Learn

about bioavailable protein dense foods, complex/simple carbohydrates, fiber, and the different types of fat. Discover which foods contain micronutrients that your body needs.

- Learn about any government programs that provide nutritional food/funding that you are eligible for.

- Everyday Lifestyle Integration/Enjoyment
  - Sit down with your spouse, roommates, family, or other relevant people and include them in the conversation about your food journey.
  - What are your flavor preferences?
  - What types of cuisine are you interested in learning to cook?
  - Who can you invite to join you on your food journey?
  - Learn and experiment with recipes and meals you enjoy that will also be more cost efficient for your household while providing the nutrients you need.
  - Figure out an eating pattern that you can commit to that works with your sleep, wake, fitness, and work schedule.
  - What is your budget for store-bought foods?
  - Learn to "shop smart" at the grocery store.

Engage

- Ancestral Foodways
  - Plant something, as much or as little as you can reasonably manage and maintain, and take very seriously the task of nurturing and growing those foods.
  - Go hunting, fishing, or trapping, following all proper spiritual and logistical protocols for respect and safety.
  - Go foraging, following the seasons and local protocols.
  - You have researched basic knowledge of tribal food sovereignty and you now attend conferences, gatherings, online trainings, or other events to bolster your knowledge.

- Nutrition/Physical Health

- Identify which foods you consider nourishing and optimal for health that you want to eat frequently, which foods you think should be approached with moderation, and which foods or substances should be completely out of your circle, antithetical to your health goals and needs.
- Observe the effects of different foods on your health, mood, spirit, energy, and so on. Become aware of how different foods make you feel. Do this both intuitively and by measurement, such as measuring blood sugar levels or tracking weight gain or loss.

- Everyday Lifestyle Integration/Enjoyment
  - You begin to cook regularly, at least one meal a day, rather than go out to eat or buy premade foods all the time.
  - You experiment with fasting periods between meals.
  - You're beginning to find out what windows of time are best for you and your family to eat.
  - You visit and begin to shop at the grocery stores or markets in your area or online that you have access to, and you go there prepared with knowledge of your established nutritional needs, budget, and familial needs.

Optimize

- Ancestral Foodways
  - You regularly hunt, fish, grow, forage, and harvest foods to feed yourself and your family.
  - You always give some of your yield to elders, those in need, those who have helped you, or any others who ask.
  - You invite loved ones, interested peers, community members, and others to join you in hunting, growing, or harvesting.
  - You have learned to minimize waste, using every part of the animal and plants that you hunt or grow.
- Nutrition/Physical Health
  - You and your family consistently follow your own ancestral foods medicine wheel.

- You have identified and regularly consult with a trusted doctor, dietician, coach, or mentor who you can talk to about your needs and food journey.
- You are comfortable with and confident shopping at the grocery stores, markets, or online shops that suit your budget, nutritional needs, etc.
- Everyday Lifestyle Integration/Enjoyment
  - You are enrolled in a benefits program that you are comfortable navigating. You have learned to cook with a variety of meats, produce, and other nutrient-dense foods that are available through this program, and you regularly offer healthy options to your family.
  - You have a well-established budget for foods that you follow, stick to, and feel comfortable with, and you have observed how this has saved you stress and worry.

INTERSECTION WITH OTHER CIRCLES

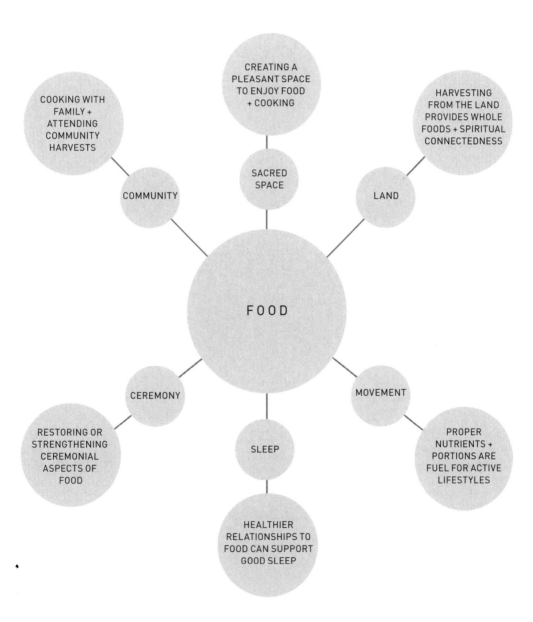

CONCLUSION
FUTURE VISIONING

The fate of our health, personal and collective, is in many ways determined by the stories we tell ourselves. Be mindful of and generous with the way you tell your own story from now on. If you tell yourself that aging is miserable, or that parenting is draining, or that movement is not for you, then that will be the case. But if you tell yourself that aging is beautiful, that parenting is magical, and that movement is for everyone, then this will be your truth.

We hope that by now, the story of Indigenous wellness has become a motivating part of your life—one that you look forward to sharing with others. If you already knew this story, fellow Indigenous people, we hope that seeing it set down in a book has brought you a sense of pride. If you didn't know this story, and if your knowledge of health and healing on this land was limited, then we hope that you now feel enlightened and inspired. We can all play our part in the continuity of this story—this rich history of living on this land in balance and reciprocity. Just as settler colonialism has caused widespread poor health and land degradation, decolonization and re-Indigenization can bring widespread healing for people and the planet. If the task of healing the world seems overwhelming, reel it in and look inward—it begins with you. Your individual pursuit of health and harmony will make an impact.

Kiowa writer N. Scott Momaday was once asked to describe the stunning natural beauty of the North American West. "It may have to be believed in order to be seen," he said.[1] Fools Crow, too, said that belief in anything precedes fruition. "How else could Wakan-Tanka and the helpers show their wonders to us?" he asked.[2] We apply this thinking to our future vision of well-being in this world. We choose to believe, with every fiber of our being, that there will be a time when the land heals, when reconnection takes place, when reciprocity reemerges, and when holistic ways of knowing become the hallmark of human life once again. When the state of the world seems bleak, we can remember the cyclical nature of the universe, and we can believe in regeneration. We ask you to join us in believing in this, if not for your own benefit, then for the benefit of those to come. Your children and descendants depend on your optimism. A world in balance is possible, but *it has to be believed in order to be seen.*

As you continue to pursue health and wholeness, and as you confront life's challenges, big and small, let these Seven Circles of Wellness be your template for returning to balance, for taking action, for remembering your power, and for remaining rooted and present in the real world. You are a vessel, a hollow bone, for good to work through. You can honor your life and attract peace and prosperity through the art of self-mastery. You can break intergenerational cycles of trauma, you can reject nihilism, and you can make a meaningful difference in the story of well-being that your children, and their children, will tell. This can be known as the era when things began to heal again.

Beyond your personal wellness journey, there are systemic changes to be made. We look forward to a time when the Seven Circles of Wellness, or holistic models like it, once again become the standard, not the radical. In industries like health care, food, and fitness, and in fields like education and government, we hope that more and more leaders will begin to take well-rounded approaches to designing systems, products, and services that incorporate and interconnect all of the Seven Circles of Wellness. We know that our ancestors lived well by keeping each of these areas centered in their lives. We must learn from and live by their knowledge.

To our Indigenous readers, friends, family, youth, and colleagues, we have seen the work that you are doing in encouraging these lifeways for our people and re-incorporating these teachings for our communities. Remember that the invaluable parts of our culture such as languages, ceremonies, songs, and foodways all maintain a symbiotic relationship to our health. When our health is good, we can more effectively and efficiently memorize songs, pass down oral traditions, grow and hunt our foods, dance in ceremonies, raise our babies, take care of our lands, and so on. And when we engage in all of these processes, our health is made even better. As we continue to feed this spirit of healing, the spirit of healing will nourish us in return.

ACKNOWLEDGMENTS
FROM BOTH OF US

We feel immensely fortunate to be represented by Jenny Stephens, our agent at Sterling Lord Literistic, who has been an impeccable advocate and a patient teacher throughout this whole process—which, as first-time authors, has been quite daunting at times. We are equally thrilled to have been teamed with our brilliant editor, Anna Paustenbach at HarperOne. That she has so completely understood and shared our vision has meant the world to us. We are also grateful to every other person at HarperCollins and Harper-One who has played a role in bringing this book to life, including Laina Adler, Sun Paik, and Adrian Morgan.

To all of the Indigenous Nations we have visited over the course of our lives and our work together, your customs of warm welcoming and your generosity with your teachings have had a significant influence on the concepts shared in this book.

To our family of colleagues at the Native Wellness Institute, we are forever grateful to have been nurtured and mentored by you over the years. The spirit of your work, and the prayers and experiences we have shared with you, are intimately woven through these pages.

THOSH

When we first found out this book was a go, I cried in happiness that I would be able to witness one of Chelsey's dreams come true. I do not take for granted how fortunate we are to have the opportunity to share what we know about living a good way of life with the world. Above all, I am happy that this book will live as a resource for our children, and all children for seven generations to come.

I am grateful to our daughters for teaching us what healing and happiness are truly about. We've realized that all of the obstacles we've overcome and all of the life teachings we've picked up along the way have led up to the moment of us becoming parents. So thank you, Alo and Westyn, for choosing us to be yours.

I give many thanks to my parents for instilling in me the teachings that have kept me well on my journey. I appreciate you, Mom, for your tireless efforts in raising us. You've always taught us about compassion and empathy through your actions. I strive to be just like you in that way. To Dad, I have so much gratitude for the years you've demonstrated what real fatherhood is all about. Every day as a father I remember the good lifeways you raised us with, and I try to pass it on to the girls. The love each of you fostered in me continues to grow and shape my own family life.

Thank you to ñ-kak, Gramma Gretta, and all of my uncles and aunties who've helped raise me. Thank you to my relatives who've traveled on to s'ialig veco (spirit world). Grampa Andy, Gramma Bobby, ñ-vikolbat Ben and Cecelia, Aunt B, Dovey, Steven, and others. Thank you for your unworldly guidance. Thank you to Chelsey's family for your constant love and support.

To my community On Akimel O'Odham jeved and the entire O'odham hemeckam (O'odham nations), this book is a reflection of the love and honor you've shown and the sense of belonging and purpose that you've fostered in me.

And finally, to my love, Chelsey, it is my truest honor to be walking alongside you in this world and during this time. My heart is forever yours. Let's continue this journey and see what other great things we can contribute to the world.

CHELSEY

I did most of my writing over the course of a pandemic that kept us all quite homebound, often restless. Office hours were between 8 p.m. and 2 a.m., sitting upright on my half of a twin bed, typing as softly as possible hoping not to wake the newborn baby who slept and grew by my side. Between these late-night work sessions were chaotic days of diaper changes, first steps, board books, and teething for Westyn; meanwhile toddler-hood, trips to the playground, and Marvel movie marathons for Alo. The special energy that comes with being in the thick of raising babies proved very helpful in keeping our words and intentions pure. I am forever grateful to Alo Akawe and Westyn Yve for expanding my heart and centering us in love. This book is for you, and in many ways, it is also by you.

Lexi, Liz, and McCall. My funnier, wiser counterparts. I am so fortunate to be your sister, and to to have the daily counsel and support of a comedian, a psychologist, and an educator.

Mom and Pat. Your unfailing love and support has held me up and kept me moving forward every single day of my life. I simply wouldn't be where I am without you.

Dad. I am forever rooted in the spiritual ways of life that you have shown me, which have been the basis of my personal wellness journey and the essential building blocks of this book.

Grandma Dorothy, Grandpa Ed, Grandma Jeanne, Grandpa Bob, Grandma Thelma, and Grandpa Butch. I will always do my best to carry your teachings and to make you proud.

All of my relatives. Kayana, Dustyn, Maya, Cassius, Eller, Ellia, Eliza. Uncles, aunties, cousins, nieces, nephews, friends, family, and community. How fortunate I am that there are too many of you to name. Thosh's family and community, you have always welcomed me as your own. I am guided daily by the memory of my late relatives Uncle Darrell, Auntie Yvonne, and Aunt Roxanne.

I have had the good fortune of learning many good things from many wonderful teachers and professors over the years. A few of those classroom experiences marked watershed moments in my life, forever changing the way that I think, learn, and understand the world. I am especially grateful to have been a student of Mrs. Mary Pomeroy, Mr. N. Bruce Duthu, Mr. Dale Turner, and Mr. Colin G. Calloway.

Finally, Thosh. I am so happy to spend my days and years with you, by your side in this work and in this life that we love so much. None of this could have been possible without your ever-flowing creativity, your commitment to wellness in action, and your very special way of bringing good people and good ideas together through your healing, radiant energy. Maybe the most amazing thing about you is that you truly walk in a way that honors your name, *Sun*.

NOTES

Introduction

1. Wilma Mankiller, *Every Day Is a Good Day: Reflections by Contemporary Indigenous Women*, memorial ed. (Golden, CO: Fulcrum, 2011), xxix.
2. Gloria Steinem, introduction to Mankiller, *Every Day Is a Good Day*, xxv.
3. Thomas E. Mails, *Fools Crow: Wisdom and Power* (San Francisco: Council Oak Books), 30–39.
4. Mails, *Fools Crow*, 40.
5. Luther Standing Bear, *Land of the Spotted Eagle* (Lincoln: Univ. of Nebraska Press, 2006), 20.
6. Paula Braveman, "Health Disparities and Health Equity: Concepts and Measurement," *Annual Review of Public Health 27* (April 2006): 167–94; WHO, 2011.
7. James N. Weinstein, Amy Geller, Yamrot Negussie, and Alina Baciu, eds., *Communities in Action: Pathways to Health Equity*, Consensus Study Report (Washington, DC: National Academies Press, 2017), available at https://www.ncbi.nlm.nih.gov/books/NBK425848/.
8. Cristine Urquhart, Fran Jasiura, and BC Provincial Mental Health and Substance Use Planning Council TIP Advisory Team, "Trauma-Informed Practice Guide," May 2013, 6–7, https://bc cewh.bc.ca/wp-content/uploads/2012/05/2013_TIP-Guide.pdf.
9. Benedict Carey, "Can We Really Inherit Trauma?," *New York Times*, December 10, 2018, https://www.nytimes.com/2018/12/10/health/mind-epigenetics-genes.html.
10. Shawn Ginwright, "The Future of Healing: Shifting from Trauma Informed Care to Healing Centered Engagement," May 31, 2018, https://ginwright.medium.com/the-future-of-healing -shifting-from-trauma-informed-care-to-healing-centered-engagement-634f557ce69c.
11. Audre Lorde, *A Burst of Light: And Other Essays* (Mineola, New York: Ixia Press, 2017), 130.

Chapter 1: Movement

1. Albert White Hat, "Lakota Health and Culture, Week 8 Part 2," YouTube, sintegleskatube (Sinte Gleska University), October 9, 2012, https://www.youtube.com/watch?v=fY3DJdkYzQs.
2. Charles Eastman, *From the Deep Woods to Civilization: Chapters in the Autobiography of an Indian*, (Lincoln and London: Bison Books / University of Nebraska Press, 1977), 1, 67–68, 111–115.
3. John Branch, "Two Hopi Traditions: Running and Winning," *New York Times*, November 4, 2015, https://www.nytimes.com/2015/11/05/sports/hopi-high-school-cross-country-running .html.
4. Larry Schwartz, "No Limits," ESPN.com, http://www.espn.com/sportscentury/features /00194728.html; "Top N. American Athletes of the Century," ESPN.com, https://www.espn .com/sportscentury/athletes.html.
5. Thomas Kaplan, "Iroquois Defeated by Passport Dispute," *New York Times*, July 16, 2010, https://www.nytimes.com/2010/07/17/sports/17lacrosse.html.
6. Ka'nhehsí:io Deer, "Supporters Challenge Iroquois Nationals' Exclusion from 2022 World Games," CBC News, July 24, 2020, https://www.cbc.ca/news/indigenous/supporters-challenge -iroquois-nationals-exclusion-from-2022-world-games-1.5662381.

7. "Community Support and Engagement," Jordan Marie Daniel, accessed January 17, 2022, https://www.jordanmariedaniel.com/community.

8. Rising Hearts, https://www.risinghearts.org.

9. Loren Kantor, "Phil Jackson's Spiritual Approach to Coaching in the NBA," Buzzer Beater, September 14, 2020, https://medium.com/buzzer-beater/phil-jacksons-spiritual-approach-to-coaching-in-the-nba-a14d249fc91c.

10. Dana Kleinjan, "Movement Matters: The Importance of Incorporating Movement in the Classroom," Master's thesis, Northwestern College, 2020; "The Mental Health Benefits of Movement," Mental Health in the Workplace, accessed January 18, 2022, https://www.mentalhealthintheworkplace.co.uk/the-mental-health-benefits-of-movement/; Heidi Godman, "Regular Exercise Changes the Brain to Improve Memory, Thinking Skills," Harvard Health Publishing, Harvard Medical School, April 9, 2014, https://www.health.harvard.edu/blog/regular-exercise-changes-brain-improve-memory-thinking-skills-201404097110.

11. Thomas E. Mails, *Fools Crow: Wisdom and Power* (San Francisco: Council Oak Books), 85–86.

12. "Mental Health Benefits of Movement."

13. Annie Murphy Paul, *The Extended Mind: The Power of Thinking Outside the Brain* (Boston: Houghton Mifflin Harcourt, 2021), 68–71.

14. US Environmental Protection Agency, "Indoor Air Quality," Report on the Environment, https://www.epa.gov/report-environment/indoor-air-quality.

15. Charles Eastman, "What Can the Out-of-Doors Do for Our Children?," *Education: A Monthly Magazine* 41 (September–June 1921): 599–600.

16. Amelia Nierenberg, "Classrooms Without Walls, and Hopefully Covid," *New York Times*, last updated November 20, 2020, https://www.nytimes.com/2020/10/27/us/outdoor-classroom-design.html.

17. Kate Bradshaw, "Covid-19 Transformed the World of Outdoor Education. Here's What Local Leaders Say Has Changed," Palo Alto Online, May 17, 2021, https://paloaltoonline.com/news/2021/05/17/covid-19-transformed-the-world-of-outdoor-education-heres-what-local-leaders-say-has-changed.

18. Charles Eastman, "What Can the Out-of-Doors Do for Our Children?," Education Volume XLI, September 1920–June 1921, 602; https://play.google.com/store/books/details?id=nSc5AAAAMAAJ&rdid=book-nSc5AAAAMAAJ&rdot=1.

Chapter 2: Land

1. Dan Buettner, *The Blue Zones: 9 Lessons for Living Longer from the People Who've Lived the Longest*, 2nd ed. (Washington, DC: National Geographic, 2008).

2. Jessica Hicks, "This Is What 5, 10, and 20 Minutes of Spending Time Outside Can Do for Your Well-Being," Thrive Global, February 21, 2020, https://thriveglobal.com/stories/nature-spending-time-outside-benefits-few-minutes/.

Chapter 3: Community

1. Bob Avenson, "Five Ways to Enhance Social Connection," Ornish Living, accessed January 2022, https://www.ornish.com/zine/increase-social-connection/.

2. Language translation provided by Art Wilson, Tohono O'odham nation.
3. "Tom Porter, Haudenosaunee Peacemaking Stories," YouTube, OYA Online, accessed January 2022, https://www.youtube.com/watch?v=Tv0PWtv4FqE&t=235s.
4. "Our Philosophy: We Observe and Value the Seven Grandfather Teachings," Leech Lake Tribal College, accessed January 2022, https://www.lltc.edu/about-us/our-philosophy/.
5. Valerie Strauss, "How Are America's Public Schools Really Doing?," *Washington Post*, October 15, 2018, https://www.washingtonpost.com/education/2018/10/15/how-are-americas-public-schools-really-doing/.

Chapter 4: Ceremony

1. Carol Schaefer, *Grandmothers Counsel the World: Women Elders Offer Their Vision for Our Planet* (Boulder, CO: Trumpeter, 2006), 15.
2. Tate quoted in Michelle Wallace, *Black Popular Culture* (Seattle: Bay Press, 1992), 13–15.
3. Esther Perel and Mary Alice Miller, "Rituals for Healthy Relationships at Every Stage," *Esther Perel Blog*, accessed January 2022, https://www.estherperel.com/blog/rituals-for-healthy-relationships.
4. Terri Suntjens, "Ceremony and the Brain with Dr. Michael Yellow Bird," *2 Crees in a Pod*, June 14, 2020, https://anchor.fm/terri-suntjens/episodes/Ceremony-and-the-Brain-with-Dr-Michael-Yellow-Bird-ef0ib2.
5. Bianca Baker, "Why Everything Is Getting Louder," *The Atlantic*, November 2019, https://www.theatlantic.com/magazine/archive/2019/11/the-end-of-silence/598366/.
6. Perel and Miller, "Rituals for Healthy Relationships."
7. Stephanie Mansour, "Start Your Day with Breathing Exercises for Stress Relief," CNN Health, last updated July 26, 2021, https://www.cnn.com/2021/07/23/health/morning-breathing-exercises-stress-relief-wellness/index.html.
8. This quotation is attributed to Gen. Richard H. Pratt, who was founder of an Indian school in Pennsylvania. See Kyle L. Simonson and Gavin M. Nadeau, "Truth and Reconciliation: 'Kill the Indian, and Save the Man,'" *Native Times*, December 3, 2016, https://www.nativetimes.com/archives/46-life/commentary/14059-truth-and-reconciliationkill-the-indian-and-save-the-man.
9. Lee Irwin, "Freedom, Law and Prophecy: A Brief History of Native American Religious Resistance," *American Indian Quarterly* 21, No. 1, Special Issue: To Hear the Eagles Cry: Contemporary Themes in Native American Spirituality: Part III: Historical Reflections (Winter 1997): 35–36, https://www.jstor.org/stable/1185587?saml_data=eyJzYW1sVG9rZW4iOiJiMjZlYjlmOS00MGI4LTQ4OGItOTI4NC0yNmEzMGY4OWY3OTIiLCJpbnN0aXR1dGlvbklkcyI6WyI2ZDg0MDkyYS1mMDBlLTRlZTQtOTYwMC1lNzJiY2VlNjdhMTQiXX0&seq=2.
10. Myles Hudson, "Wounded Knee Massacre," Encyclopedia Britannica, accessed April 12, 2022, https://www.britannica.com/event/Wounded-Knee-Massacre.

Chapter 5: Sacred Space

1. Irem Sultana, Arshad Ali, and Ifra Iftikhar, "Effects of Horror Movies on Psychological Health of Youth," *GMCR, Global Mass Communication Review* 6, no. 1 (Winter 2021), https://gmcrjournal.com/papers/xFc88IkFQ7.pdf.

2. Emilie Le Beau Lucchesi, "The Unbearable Heaviness of Clutter," *New York Times*, January 3, 2019, https://www.nytimes.com/2019/01/03/well/mind/clutter-stress-procrastination-psychology.html.

3. Carol Schaefer, *Grandmothers Counsel the World: Women Elders Offer Their Vision for Our Planet* (Boulder, CO: Trumpeter, 2006), 79.

4. "Social Media Fact Sheet," Pew Research Center, April 7, 2021, https://www.pewresearch.org/internet/fact-sheet/social-media/.

5. Helen Lee Bouygues, "Social Media Is a Public Health Crisis. Let's Treat It like One," *U.S. News & World Report*, July 20, 2021, https://www.usnews.com/news/health-news/articles/2021-07-20/social-media-is-a-public-health-crisis.

6. Nick Dauk, "Is Internet Addiction a Growing Problem?," BBC News, October 25, 2021, https://www.bbc.com/news/business-58979895.

7. Spencer Hulse, "Companies Pushing Toward the Metaverse," *Grit Daily*, February 7, 2022, https://gritdaily.com/companies-pushing-toward-the-metaverse/; Phil Reed, "Will the Metaverse Impact Mental Health?," *Psychology Today*, October 27, 2021, https://www.psychologytoday.com/us/blog/digital-world-real-world/202110/will-the-metaverse-impact-mental-health.

Chapter 6: Sleep

1. "Brain Basics: Understanding Sleep," National Institute of Neurological Disorders and Stroke, last updated August 13, 2019, https://www.ninds.nih.gov/Disorders/Patient-Caregiver-Education/understanding-Sleep#2.

2. "Sleep, Learning, and Memory," Healthy Sleep, Harvard Medical School Division of Sleep Medicine, last reviewed December 18, 2007, https://healthysleep.med.harvard.edu/healthy/matters/benefits-of-sleep/learning-memory.

3. "Brain Basics."

4. Excerpt from Harvey R. Colten and Bruce M. Altevogt, eds., *Sleep Disorders and Sleep Deprivation: An Unmet Public Health Problem* (Washington, DC: National Academies Press, 2006), https://pubmed.ncbi.nlm.nih.gov/20669438/.

5. "Short Sleep Duration Among US Adults," Data and Statistics: Sleep and Sleep Disorders, last reviewed May 2, 2017, https://www.cdc.gov/sleep/data_statistics.html.

6. Maureen Salamon, Medically Reviewed by Whitney Seltman, OD, "How Blue Light Affects Your Sleep," Web MD, October 3, 2020, https://www.webmd.com/sleep-disorders/sleep-blue-light.

7. Colten and Altevogt, *Sleep Disorders and Sleep Deprivation*.

8. Danielle Pacheco and Heather Wright, "Sleep and Blood Glucose Levels," Sleep Foundation, last updated March 11, 2022, https://www.sleepfoundation.org/physical-health/sleep-and-blood-glucose-levels.

Chapter 7: Food

1. National Center for Chronic Disease Prevention and Health Promotion, "Chronic Disease Fact Sheets," Centers for Disease Control and Prevention, last reviewed May 12, 2021, https://www.cdc.gov/chronicdisease/resources/publications/fact-sheets.htm.

2. "Foods Linked to Better Brainpower," Harvard Health Publishing, Harvard Medical School, March 6, 2021, https://www.health.harvard.edu/healthbeat/foods-linked-to-better-brain power.

3. Sunghyon Kyeong, John Kim, Dae Jin Kim, Hesun Erin Kim, and Jae-Jin Kim, "Effects of Grati-tude Meditation on Neural Network Functional Connectivity and Brain-Heart Coupling," *Scien-tific Reports* 7 (2017): 5058, https://www.ncbi.nlm.nih.gov/pmc/articles/PMC5506019/.

4. "Ciolim (Cholla Buds)," San Xavier Co-Op Farm, accessed January 2022, https://www .sanxaviercoop.org/product/ciolim-cholla-buds/.

Conclusion: Future Visioning

1. *The West*, episode 1, "The People (to 1806)," a documentary film presented by Ken Burns, di-rected by Stephen Ives. Originally aired September 15, 1996, PBS, accessed 2022, Amazon Prime Video, https://www.amazon.com/Ken-Burns-West-Season-1/dp/B0090X4BUI/ref=dv _web_auth_no_re_sig?_encoding=UTF8&.

2. Thomas E. Mails, *Fools Crow: Wisdom and Power* (San Francisco: Council Oak Books), 81.